Adoptable Dog

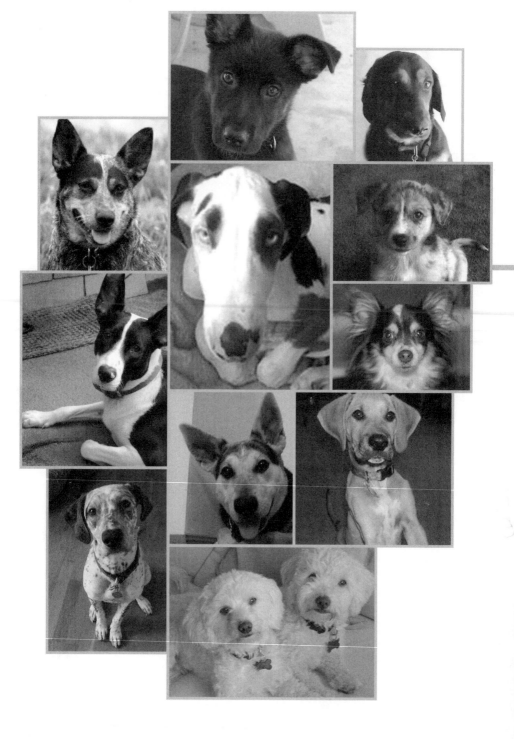

Adoptable Dog

Teaching Your Adopted Pet to Obey, Trust, and Love You

John Ross *and* Barbara McKinney

W.W. Norton & Company

New York London

Frontispiece: The dogs featured on the title-page spread are either
rescued or adopted dogs.

For information about permission to reproduce selections from this book, write to
Permissions, W. W. Norton & Company, Inc., 500 Fifth Avenue, New York, NY 10110

Manufacturing by Maple-Vail Book Manufacturing Group
Book design by Lovedog Studio
Production manager: Julia Druskin

LIBRARY OF CONGRESS CATALOGING–IN–PUBLICATION DATA

Ross, John.
Adoptable dog : teaching your adopted pet to obey, trust, and love you / by John
Ross and Barbara McKinney.— 1st ed.
p. cm.
Includes bibliographical references (p.   ) and index.
ISBN 0-393-05079-3 (hardcover)
1. Dogs—Training. 2. Dogs—Behavior.
I. McKinney, Barbara. II. Title.
SF431 .R648 2003
636.7'0835—dc21
2002013395

W. W. Norton & Company, Inc., 500 Fifth Avenue, New York, N.Y. 10110
www.wwnorton.com

W. W. Norton & Company Ltd., Castle House, 75/76 Wells Street, London W1T 3QT

1 2 3 4 5 6 7 8 9 0

This book is dedicated to
those who devote their careers
and their hearts
to helping adopted dogs.
You are making the world
a better place.
Thank you.

Contents

Preface

As a **person dedicated** to teaching people how to train their dogs, I feel that writing books is a natural extension of what I do. *Adoptable Dog* may be my most significant book yet, because it covers a vast population of dogs that have been ignored by almost all dog authors in the past.

The United States Humane Society estimates that 4 to 5 million dogs enter shelters each year. Sadly, about half of them are euthanized. What happens to the other 2.5 million dogs? They are adopted. This means that at any given time, assuming an average ten-year life span as an adoptee, 25 million adopted dogs are living in this country. That is a substantial part of the United States' entire population of pet dogs, about 62 million. *Adoptable Dog* speaks to the millions of dog owners out there who need guidance for living compatibly with their adopted pet.

I have to admit that the idea of this book did not immediately inspire me. This is because Barbara McKinney and I both have been purebred dog enthusiasts for many years—she with her beloved Labradors and I with my field-bred sporting dogs. Although I had adopted a couple of dogs over the years, I was not deeply involved with shelters and their work.

As we searched for new writing ideas, we concluded that a book about adopted dogs was not needed for educating animal rescue workers or adoption counselors. There are thousands of dedicated people who are experts in this field. They know more than I do about catching strays, evaluating age and health, screening adoption candidates, and even rehabilitating some undesirables to give them a chance at adoption. I tip my baseball hat to their wonderful efforts. Dog lovers everywhere owe them our profound thanks.

My expertise is not in providing assistance to these dedicated animal rescue workers. It is in helping owners with their new dogs—whether they are puppies, adolescents, or adults. My training programs give people the skills needed to communicate with and to train their dogs of any breed or age. However, I recognized long ago that adopted dogs often have special needs. I have incorporated unique material into my training programs for this vast dog population. In fact, I have been teaching these skills to adopted dogs and their owners for thirty years now. This is the focus of *Adoptable Dog*.

It is my conviction that successful training will virtually guarantee that an adopted dog will become a lifetime family member. I have observed all too often that without proper training, the adopted dog becomes stuck in a revolving door of banishment from his pack. It is traumatic to a dog to be given away, and the trauma is intensified each time it happens. This book's goal is to help keep adopted dogs with their new owners. I hope that you find it useful—and that your adopted dog has found with you a lifelong home and family.

—John Ross

Acknowledgments

WE GRATEFULLY ACKNOWLEDGE the many dog owners and dogs who contributed to this book. Helping with our photographs were Nancy Scully and Max, Jill Wattles and Thumper (the Jumper), Helen Savill with Jet and Winnie, Jackie MacMullen and Missy, Alfred Stebbins and Buddy, Lois Hollinger and Hollie, Marie George, Peggy Dyer, Cara Anderson, and the Roberts family: Tyrone, Susan, Sara, Tyler, and Emma (the dog).

Special thanks to our photographer, Joann Wilson of Wilson Photography in Stuart, Florida.

The staff at the Humane Society of the Treasure Coast (Florida) was welcoming to us in every way during this book project. Wally Burleson, Executive Director; Ed Wilson, Shelter Manager; and especially Helen Savill, Director of Humane Education, opened their doors and their hearts to us to share behind-the-scenes information about adoptable dogs. They represent animal welfare work at its finest.

Julie Starkweather has our eternal gratitude for breeding our beloved Labradors, Byron and Bentley. But her breed rescue work puts her in a special category of amazing. Thank you, Julie, for sharing your wisdom and stories—and for making a big difference in so many dogs' lives.

Thank you to our veterinary consultant, the great Dr. Chuck Noonan, Animal Doctor of Weston (Connecticut), for his medical expertise. Dr. Chuck and his staff are always just a phone call away.

It seems that all our dog books somehow find their way into the hands of our favorite editor, Bob Weil. Thank you, Bob (and feisty little Tucker), for inspiration, guidance, and some great dog stories. This book was helped into reality by Bob's assistant, Jason Baskin, and our most capable and supportive agent, Cynthia Cannell.

Part One

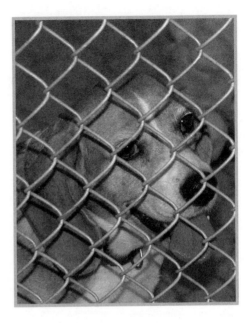

Adopting the Right Dog

A kennel full of sad-eyed homeless dogs is enough to melt any dog lover's heart. But you can't take them all home. Here are important guidelines for finding the right dog for you.

Chapter 1

Why Adopt?
The Pros and Cons

IN A SENSE, every dog is adopted. Even an eight-week-old puppy leaves its mother and littermates to be taken in by its new human owners.

But that is not what we mean by "adopted dogs." Adopted dogs are castoffs. They started life in one setting, the newborn period with mother dog and her owner, and next they moved into their first home on their own to live with a human family. Then for one reason or another, they had to leave that home.

Some dogs move in and out of several homes before finding one that lasts. Realistically, few dogs get that many chances. Dogs that cannot fit in are usually euthanized without ever finding an owner willing to make a lifelong commitment. I hope this book will help change that.

Dogs are put up for adoption for all sorts of reasons. Many are strays, picked up by animal control officers or turned in by someone who was concerned for the dog's safety. All too frequently, owners give up their dogs when they are no longer able—or willing—to care for them. An owner's death or arrest can send a dog to a shelter, but so can a court order if the dog is suffering from abuse or neglect. Dogs such as retired racing greyhounds often can be adopted, too.

Adoptable dogs come in a great many varieties—not determined by breed so much as by their individual history. They may be young, old, or in between. They may have lived in a busy household with kids, cats, and other dogs, or they may have spent many quiet years with a senior citizen and never met any children or other animals. Adopted dogs may have been loved and cherished (a rarity!) or painfully abused. They may have roamed urban streets, lived outdoors on a ranch, or never left a small suburban condo. They may have fought other dogs for scraps of food or become painfully obese from overindulgence. You get the idea. Adoptable dogs don't have much in common except that they all need homes.

Giving a second chance to a homeless dog can be a wonderful, fulfilling experience, both for you and the dog. I have met many happy owners and their devoted adopted dogs over the past thirty years. Truthfully, some adoptions do not work out well. Chapter 16 describes what to do when the best efforts fail. But there are a lot of good reasons to adopt a dog. Here are some important ones.

Adopting Is Cheaper Than Buying

Purebred dogs from reputable breeders cost hundreds, often thousands, of dollars. Part of what you are paying for is predictability. A puppy from a Doberman pinscher breeder really is a Doberman. It will grow into an adult that conforms to certain breed standards, such as size, weight, type of coat, color, etc. Within a certain range, its temperament and instincts will be like those of other Dobermans—not like those of collies or pugs or Chihuahuas.

Your payment to a breeder also gives you some level of assurance about the dog's physical and mental soundness. Don't misunderstand! There are plenty of disreputable breeders who will put a high price tag on any puppy they can manage to produce. But a good breeder takes the time and trouble to produce great puppies. He or she studies the traits and histories of the breeding stock. With the help of a veterinarian and various medical tests, the breeder evaluates the sire and the dam. He or she checks for healthy bone structure, eyesight, hearing, teeth alignment, and risk for disease, such as epilepsy and diabetes.

A responsible breeder provides good prenatal care to the mother dog, helping her to give birth safely. Each puppy gets early veterinary care, including vaccinations and wormings. The puppies get a clean, warm environment in which to play, sleep, and eat. A good breeder also keeps the pups with the mother dog until they are old enough to go home with their new owners.

It takes a lot of effort to breed high-quality dogs. For the most part, the high cost of a good breeder's puppies reflects the time, expertise, expense, and care that is put into each breeding.

What does all this have to do with adopting dogs? In a way, everything, because you cannot expect to get any of the above when you adopt. There is no guarantee of health screenings on the dog's parents or prenatal care for the mother dog. Depending on where you get the dog, he may not have had veterinary checkups and vaccinations. These things often are left to chance when you adopt.

That's not to say that well-bred dogs never show up at local shelters or get listed in the newspaper for adoption. They do, of course. But you are not getting the same assurance as when you give top dollar to a reputable breeder.

Is that okay with you? Only you can answer that question. Great, healthy dogs can be found in all sorts of places, including the local animal shelter. Finding one is up to you.

So yes, adopting a dog is cheaper than buying one—as long as the adopted dog is healthy and trainable. A few hefty bills from the veterinarian and a dozen payments to a "doggie behavior therapist" will quickly consume any savings you enjoyed when you got the dog. So be prepared to choose an adopted dog wisely. Chapter 4 will show you how.

You Don't Have to Deal with Puppyhood

This is a great reason to adopt a dog. Puppyhood is a lot of work. The time and energy required to housebreak, supervise, and train a young dog are by no means minimal. I tell my clients that a new puppy is almost like having a human baby in the house. There are great joys, but it is also very demanding.

Puppies are immature dogs until they are about two years old. Especially during their first year of life, puppies can be rambunctious

goofballs. Without supervision and training, they will urinate and defecate around the house, jump all over visitors, chew rugs, steal food, bite
people, dig up the yard, and bark too much. It is up to the owner to
teach the puppy to behave.

An adult dog may not do any of those things. Of course, it is possible that you end up with the proverbial wolf in sheep's clothing—that
is, a nice-looking adult dog with all of the undesirable behaviors of a
puppy! And to make matters worse, these undesirable behaviors are not
changed as easily in adult dogs as they are in puppies. Puppies have not
been alive long enough to have deeply seated bad habits. Adult dogs
have. A two-year-old dog that barks nonstop and pees in the house has
probably been doing these things for two years. Changing these
behaviors in an adult dog is not impossible, but it will take a lot more
time and work than it would to train a puppy.

So, you should choose an adopted adult dog wisely. Otherwise your
goal of avoiding the training and the constant supervision that a puppy
requires will not be realized.

It is certainly possible that you may find an adult dog that is well
trained. Housebreaking and unwanted chewing are not an issue.
Greeting people calmly and without biting them is no problem.
Neither are digging and excessive barking. If you find a healthy, adoptable dog like this, go for it! You have probably found a winner.

Everybody Loves a Mutt

I certainly do. The random mixing of standard breeds has produced
some amazing, unique dogs. I have known quite a few. And I would
never advocate for a world without them. Mixed-breed dogs are the
spice of life in the dog world. They keep it from being overrun by the
kennel club set, where only properly registered, purebred individuals
are deemed to have value.

A lot of adopted dogs, especially those from shelters and pounds, are
mixed breeds. They are often the result of unintended matings.
Someone's roaming male Labrador followed his nose to the home of
a female beagle in heat. The result? "Beagle-adors." A few puppies are
given to friends or neighbors and the rest end up at the pound. (It's no

Is a Dog (Any Dog) Right for You?

Your odds for a successful adoption depend partly on the dog you choose. But success depends on you, too. Are you ready to be a good dog owner? Answer these questions to help you know for sure.

✳ Are you enthusiastic? Do other members of your household agree to adopting a dog?

✳ Are you prepared for a long-term commitment?

✳ Do you have a dog-friendly house and yard? (See Chapter 5.)

✳ Are you able and willing to pay for health care? essential supplies? obedience training?

✳ Will you work to resolve behavioral problems?

✳ Will you adjust your household routines and priorities so that the dog's needs are met?

✳ Will you provide social interaction and teach good manners so that others will enjoy being around your dog?

An unreserved "yes" to all these questions is essential before you add a dog to your family. Adopting a dog is not a casual decision that can be undone without consequences. Think through your own readiness and then adopt—but only when you are prepared to do it right.

wonder that animal shelters are such strong advocates of spaying and neutering. They see a lot of puppy dumping.)

But our emphasis is not on those eight-week-old puppies; it's on adolescent and adult mixed-breed dogs. Why are there so many of them in the pounds? My theory is that most mixed-breed dogs are produced by irresponsible owners. A good owner doesn't *let* his intact male roam around the neighborhood or allow an in-heat female to be unsupervised for even a moment. In fact, good owners typically don't even have fertile pets. They believe in spaying and neutering and have made sure that their dogs (and cats) have had this surgery.

But breeding accidents do happen. When the mother dog is given good prenatal care and is helped to deliver safely and veterinary care is given to her puppies, the results can be perfectly fine. So a mixed-breed dog is not, by definition, an undesirable choice. In fact, some people feel that "mutts" are healthier, stronger, and longer-lived than purebreds.

Mixed-breed dogs can be fun to own. They have a uniqueness that reflects the random mixing of all kinds of dog traits. I once knew an adorable small German-shepherd-type dog with three-inch Corgi-size legs. I have known Labs with chow chow fur, huskies with shepherd faces, and poodles with big golden retriever heads. It has been fun for me, over the years, to see these combinations and meet some unique dogs. Occasionally I'll ask the owner, "What's in *him*?" More than once I've been told, "We have no idea. Even the vet can't guess." As I said, mutts are the spice of life.

Surprise, Surprise

Sometimes adopted dogs can bring unfortunate surprises. These could include an undiagnosed disease, an undiagnosed pregnancy (!), or early death if the dog's age is underestimated. Careful screening of your potential dog by adoption counselors and a veterinarian will help you minimize the chance for these problems.

Puppies and adolescent dogs may surprise you by growing into something different from what you expect. They may look like minia-ture adults, but they might mature into a dog that is quite different in size, shape, and color. Those cute, short legs may never get any longer. That fluffy, soft coat might shed and be replaced by sleek, stiff fur. That big, oversized head may always look somewhat big and oversized.

However, some surprises can be fun. If you tend to focus on what's *inside* a dog, such as personality, trainability, and companionship, an adoptable dog of any age is a good candidate for you.

There Are Too Many Homeless Dogs in the World

This is a great reason to adopt a dog. Millions of healthy, wonderful dogs are euthanized every year because no one wants them. Putting these animals to death—because we humans have not acted responsibly—is immoral, in my opinion. What a powerful indicator of how ignorant and wasteful we can be.

I would like to think that sometime in this new millennium every litter of puppies will be planned and every dog will have a home. Until then, I cannot improve on the current adoption system. Our humane organizations, local shelters, and breed rescue groups are working to solve a big, ugly problem. If you are helping the cause by adopting a dog, I believe that you are a special person and that you are making the world a better place. On behalf of all dogs and dog lovers everywhere, thank you!

Now, if you are ready to adopt a dog, let's find you the right one.

Chapter 2

What Are You Looking For?

ONE OF THE BEST WAYS to have a successful experience with adopting a dog is to know yourself: what you like and don't like, what you can handle and can't handle, what your family will or will not enjoy, what's appropriate for your lifestyle—and what is not.

Ideally, you should start the adoption process by thinking through your requirements before you go dog shopping. This is not always realistic, of course. Emergency situations, such as a relative's death or a neighbor's move, may place an adopted dog in your lap. If you are on a waiting list with a local pound, a sudden overflow of homeless animals in their facility may result in a phone call request to *please* take a dog now. Or you may have stopped by the humane society to drop off a donation, and now Scruffy is riding home with you in the backseat.

Barring such unexpected situations, take time to plan your adoption. It will be well worth the effort. Start by thinking about what sort of "features" you want in a dog, such as big versus little, old versus young. Think about what you can reasonably handle: mostly trained versus not at all trained, healthy versus unhealthy. Think about your family members and what they like, too. These are some of the many issues to consider in finding the right adoptable dog. This chapter will help you sort them all out.

Your ultimate goal should be to find a dog that is a great match for you, your family, your home, and your lifestyle. This will increase ten-fold—maybe a hundredfold—the chances that your adopted dog will come to stay.

If an adopted dog already lives in your home, this chapter will help you better understand your dog's fit into your home. It may reveal problem areas that require your attention so that you and your dog can improve on your relationship. Perhaps it will even give you the confidence and inspiration to open your home to another adoptable canine friend.

Health Considerations

Are you able and willing to care for an adopted dog with known health problems? These may be as minor as an odd-growing toenail that needs special trimming or waxy ears that need frequent cleaning. They could also be as major as canine diabetes, which requires daily insulin injections, or early kidney disease in which the dog only has a year to live.

Some health problems are fixable, if you are willing to go through the process and bear the expense. A parasite infestation, such as a case of hookworm or a coat full of fleas, can be overcome with a veterinarian's help. So can mange (an itchy skin condition), tooth or gum disease, infected wounds, and the like. Although an adopted dog may be virtually "free to a good home," the costs of owning a dog with health issues can quickly add up.

So sort through your feelings and capabilities on this subject. Certainly it is true that *any* dog could develop health problems at any time during its life, which the owner must attend to. But most of us expect to get some years of healthful enjoyment from our pets. Don't adopt an animal with an illness if you are not truly willing and able to provide appropriate care right from the start.

Physical Imperfections

These are healthy dogs with disabilities: a missing eye, an amputated leg, two-thirds of a tail. I have known dogs with these conditions. They are great dogs! Fortunately, dogs don't have ego involvement in their

Pampered Pooch vs. Street Waif

Do you envision your adopted dog as a bedraggled, homeless wanderer, suddenly transported into a wonderful life of regular meals, a warm bed, and a loving family? Or are you looking for a pampered pooch that already knows—and expects—the finer things in a dog's life?

An adopted dog's background will certainly influence its adjustment into your home. Surprisingly, the homeless wanderers usually do extremely well. They are familiar with the ups and downs of life, and they take change in stride. Most of them have connected with a variety of different people over the years, and they are perfectly content to let you be their next friend. They might have liked the roaming life a little *too* much, so be prepared with secure fencing in your yard and a strong grip on the leash.

On the other hand, Fifi the Fluffy may have never known a day outside her one owner's loving care. When that longtime owner dies or becomes hospitalized, Fifi must face change for the first time in her life. Dogs like this may have a really rough time throughout the adoption process. If Fifi ends up in a shelter or pound, the stresses of living there with many different caretakers can be overwhelming. So can the task of adjusting to a new home and family. Once Fifi is settled in, she will likely be a great, devoted pet. Just be prepared to give her a little extra time. A predictable daily routine helps, too. This will allow her to find familiarity in the new environment and, eventually, to accept it as her own.

appearance. They know that they are just as good as all the other dogs on the block.

But humans do have egos, which can influence their opinions about dogs. If you won't feel good about an imperfect pet, you would be wise not to adopt one. Keep in mind, though, that such dogs can be quite interesting. I used to tell people that my one-eyed black Lab, Byron, lost his eye rescuing me during a seaplane crash. It wasn't true, of course, but it got some laughs and helped people to look at Byron affectionately, which he always returned in kind.

Age

In most cases, the younger the dog the better the results with obedience training. This takes some qualification. Five-week-old puppies should not be adopted. The best place for young puppies is with their mother. But after they reach seven or eight weeks of age and are in good health, adoption into a new home is fine.

As I stated earlier in this book, initial puppy adoptions are not the focus of *Adoptable Dog*. However, some relatively young dogs *are* given up for secondary adoption, and their new owners will certainly need the guidelines provided in these chapters.

The advantage of adopting a young dog is that it has not been around long enough to develop deeply seated bad habits. The dog may have *plenty* of unwanted behaviors, but these behaviors are not as

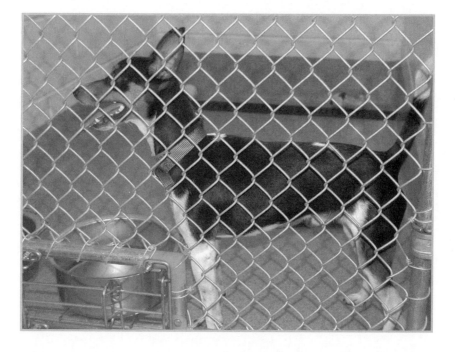

Think about the "dog traits" that are a good fit for you and your home. This small terrier has short hair and a lively personality. Don't pick him if you want a big, furry couch potato.

resistant to change as the habits of a two- or three-year-old adult dog. This means that obedience training will probably be a lot easier. Of course, it also means that you will need to commit the time needed for obedience training. Don't get a young dog and expect it to magically turn into a calm, well-behaved adult. It is up to you to make that happen.

Here's an interesting question to consider on this subject: Would you rather have an out-of-control eight-month-old adolescent dog or a calm, four-year-old dog that never comes when called? Both animals will require training to overcome their problems. What are you up for: taming a rambunctious pup for the next eight to ten months or spending several years repeating the specific Come on Command training exercises? Only you can decide what is better for you.

Also there are plenty of opportunities for adopting a canine senior citizen. My observation is that most older adoptable dogs are pretty easy to live with, assuming they are in reasonably good health. Nightmarish pets—the ones that bite, run away, or snap at the kids— rarely make it to old age. They are either trained, euthanized, or exiled to the backyard, where they succumb to injury or illness and an early death.

If you like the idea of a calm dog with minimal exercise needs, an older dog may fit this niche nicely. In fact, if you are a senior citizen yourself, your lifestyle may be well matched to such a dog. The only downside I must point out is that an older dog will not be with you very long. Canine lifespans of most breeds are about twelve to fifteen years. I will be the first one to acknowledge that loving and losing a dog is a sad, heartbreaking experience. But living without one at all would be even worse. If the matchup with an appealing, elderly dog seems right for you, go for it. A few years of companionship and bliss are never a mistake.

Breed Traits

Any good reference book on dog breeds lists hundreds of known canine varieties. How can you possibly choose the best one for you? Fortunately, the breeds in most of our homes (and in most of our shel-

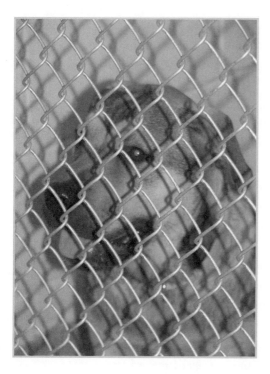

Mixed-breed dogs abound at animal shelters, but don't let the lack of a pedigree fool you. These dogs can make just as good companions as their purebred cousins.

ters) are one of just a few dozen popular breeds or mixture of these breeds. As you sort through your description of an ideal dog, consider a few broad categories to help you narrow things down.

Size   Size usually matters. Can you physically handle and comfortably house a giant breed? Then check into Great Danes, Newfoundlands, English mastiffs, Irish wolfhounds, and St. Bernards. Many dog owners shy away from adopting such big dogs. These dogs need a big enough home to move around comfortably, they are relatively expensive to feed, and they need a handler who is capable of working with a strong, heavy animal. Fortunately, many of these dogs fit the description of "gentle giant." You would be providing a needed service by taking in one of these dogs that are somewhat *un*adoptable because of their size. Breed rescue organizations might be the best place to start in seeking out a giant breed that needs a home.

Little dogs can be great fun, or yappy little terrors. One advantage with their size is that you can pick them up. You can hold them (and their muzzles) when the doorbell rings, you can carry them out to the car, and you can pick them up when they start jumping all over your grandchildren. This is one way to work around unwanted behaviors if you are not really inclined to spend the time teaching Quiet on Command, Come on Command, and Greeting People Without Jumping. Eight pounds of bratty behavior can be less problematic than eighty pounds, although a well-trained dog of any size is certainly preferable to one that needs constant hands-on management.

Coat   Grooming needs should be considered when buying or adopting any dog. Do you like brushing a dog's coat? Do you mind tufts of fur around the house? Can you afford regular trips to a groomer for clipping? Poodles, collies, wheaten terriers, and other long-haired breeds will cost you time and money for coat care. Rule out individuals with high-end grooming needs if you are not willing to provide what they require.

Barking   Some breeds are known for noise. The terriers (which I love) come to mind. So do shelties, dachshunds, and schnauzers. Drifter, my late, great Australian shepherd, also loved to bark. A dog that barks too much *for you* can be a deal-breaker.

People have very different tolerances for dog noise. So do neighbors. If you live in close proximity to others, consider carefully the barking tendencies of a potential pet. An obedience skill that I teach, called Quiet on Command, can help you manage a barker. So can several kinds of collars that create an unpleasant sensation for the dog when he barks. The bottom line is that you are responsible for your dog's barking, whether it's a lot or a little. Be prepared.

Trainability   Trainability is an important consideration with an adopted dog, especially if the dog has unwanted behaviors that you plan to train away. Some breeds, generally speaking, are easier to train than others. In one of our books, *Puppy Preschool*, we list and describe ten popular breeds that usually respond very well to training. We also describe ten breeds that are usually more of a challenge. Fortunately, adoptable dogs are not little puppies, and you do not need to rely on breed generalities to select a good pet. When you are evaluating an adolescent or adult dog for adoption, what you see is basically what you get. This means that you can evaluate the individual dog, no matter what its breed. However, try to gather as much information as possible about the dog from shelter workers, previous owners, or the veterinarian. These individuals may help you determine what kind of training effort your new dog will require.

A Quiz: What Are You Looking For?

Take this test. There are no right or wrong answers. Instead, the questions will guide you in finding an adopted dog that is a good fit for you and your household.

Be sure to have other members of your family consider these questions, too. Conflicting answers, if any, will allow you to deal with the different expectations you may have about dog ownership. Better to sort them out now than after the adoption has taken place. Remember, your number one goal is to make the adoption a success, no matter what kind of dog you choose. Answering these questions will help.

1. Do you have room to house a big dog?
2. Would you prefer a little dog that's easy to pick up?
3. Do you like to brush and groom a dog?
4. If not, can you afford regular trips to a professional groomer?
5. Do you live where a barking dog would not disturb others?
6. Are you motivated to do much obedience training?
7. Can you manage the demands of supervising a puppy?
8. Would you enjoy a few years with a calm canine senior?
9. Would you like a dog that has roamed far and wide? Or one that has known the comforts of only one home?
10. Can you afford to provide above-average veterinary care to an adopted dog with special medical needs? Are you *willing* to provide it?
11. Are you bothered by physical impairments, such as a missing eye or limb?
12. Is your household chaotic, quiet, or somewhere in between?

Input from Your Family

Unless you live alone, all of the above considerations must receive input from your family members as well. In my experience, a dog that is loved and cared for by one family member but ignored or hated by another is a dog that would be better placed with different owners. Keep in mind that dogs are pack animals. A dog views everyone in his home as his pack. A harmonious pack, in which each member feels bonded to the others, is the best scenario for dog ownership. So don't let choosing a dog become the focus of a marital feud or teenage battleground. It is not fair to the dog and may be a good indication that in the long run the adoption will not be a happy one.

Lifestyle Match

Think about the rhythms and routines of your household. Is there a lot of activity and noise? A lot of children or teenagers (or both) running around? Perhaps you work at home and have clients stopping by each day. Or you manage a store and have customers coming and going who will meet your dog. Do you travel a lot or take long summer vacations? On the other hand, you may live alone and lead a quiet life. You are at home most of the time and enjoy a short, daily walk and a good book.

The dog you adopt should be a good match for your lifestyle. For example, a shy, ten-year-old arthritic dog probably would not join in on the chaotic fun of a houseful of children. And an energetic one-year-old sporting dog might need a lot more exercise than a sedentary senior could provide. Dogs are highly adaptable creatures and can usually adjust to any loving environment. But you want the best for your pet. Be prepared to choose one that will be a good fit for you.

Almost Ready

Use as much reason and common sense as you possibly can in thinking about the right kind of adoptable dog for your home. I can almost guarantee that the minute you walk past a row of cages at the animal shelter and look into all those sweet, homeless faces, you will want to toss your carefully laid plans out the window! That's okay for some things, like the dog's age or coat, if the dog you love is otherwise still a decent match. But don't ignore all your planning efforts. Remind yourself (over and over again, if necessary) that the long-term success of the adoption is greatly influenced by getting the right fit.

Let the shelter workers or adoption supervisor help you. Share the details of your household and lifestyle and explain what you want in an adopted dog. These individuals can put the information to good use in finding you one or more dogs to consider.

I wish I could say that there are not enough adoptable dogs for every available home—and that being a little picky means that you will never find a good dog. Sadly, that's not true. Depending on the size of your community, you may have to wait awhile for a dog that matches your exact criteria to become available. But you can also go looking outside your community, and I guarantee that you will find many, many nice dogs needing homes. There are more than enough to go around.

Chapter 3

Evaluating Adoption Resources

ADOPTABLE DOGS ARE EVERYWHERE. They are as close as your city's pound or as distant as a breed rescue organization across the continent. How far you reach to adopt a dog really depends on you. Highly specific adoption requirements, such as a certain breed of a particular sex of an exact age, may require you to look farther afield. Sometimes our heartstrings are tugged long-distance when a homeless dog's tragic plight makes the news, and adoption offers pour in from across the country.

Most people seeking to adopt dogs stick close to home. That's because we rarely need to look very far to find nice dogs, especially ones that meet just a few basic requirements. "A medium-sized dog that's housebroken, good with kids, and doesn't shed too much" is a typical request, and it's a pretty easy order to fill for most adoption organizations.

One visit to your nearby humane society or pound will also show you why many people adopt locally. It's hard to resist a kennel full of homeless dogs! Almost every time I have visited a pound or humane society on "dog business," at least one appealing, bright-eyed dog has attracted my interest. If you're a dog lover, you know what I mean. After looking into a few cute canine faces, the urge to take one home can be pretty strong.

To help you find the right dog, this chapter gives an overview of adoption resources. It is not meant to advocate one kind of organization over another, but simply profiles different kinds of adoption groups and gives you tips for deciding where to go next.

Local Pounds

Many cities, towns, and counties are mandated by law to provide food and shelter to stray animals. In rural areas, this once meant putting cows and other roaming livestock into a community holding pen until the farmer could round up the missing animals. In U.S. cities, organized protection and care of abandoned animals did not even exist 150 years ago. In 1866, the ASPCA (American Society for the Prevention of Cruelty to Animals) was founded in New York City, the first organization of its kind in North America. Today, most municipalities allocate at least some resources for animal protection.

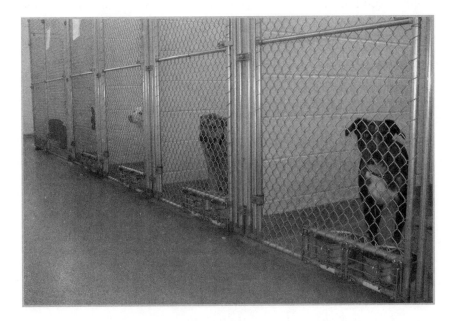

These homeless dogs are lucky to be housed in a clean, well-managed humane society where they get exercise, socialization, grooming, and veterinary care. Staff members help match new owners with the right dog, an important ingredient for a successful adoption.

Depending on the community, local pounds may be managed by police departments, county commissioners, public safety departments, etc. There is no single format for financing and managing this community service. Unfortunately, there is also no standard for quality. Some pounds are sadly underfunded, and the abandoned animals in their care may receive very little in the way of exercise, grooming, and veterinary care. Some workers are glad to ship any dog out the door to any willing owner. Happily, many publicly funded pounds do a fine job, helping animals to look and feel their best and to find permanent, appropriate homes for them.

If you go to a municipal pound in search of a dog, your job is to be especially alert and attentive to the dogs and their environment. Keep in mind that great dogs *can* be found here. You just may have to bear more of the responsibility for finding a good, healthy one yourself. There may not be adoption counselors, on-site trainers, consulting veterinarians, and a crew of loving volunteers who have cared for the animals and groomed them (literally and figuratively) for a new home. Sparky the Street Waif, sitting in the cage, may have been picked up by the dog catcher last week. It's up to you to figure out if he is healthy, emotionally sound—and the right dog for you.

If you feel particularly unsure about making a decision, consider bringing along some help. I occasionally accompany clients when they are looking over a litter of puppies. Perhaps your veterinarian will stop by the shelter and evaluate your chosen candidate. This kind of help, provided either voluntarily or for a small fee, is not an unreasonable thing to request. It can be the safety net you need if a dog in the pound seems wonderful—but you're still not sure.

Humane Societies

I have a lot of good things to say about humane societies, especially those that are well funded and well managed. Not only do they shelter and place abandoned animals, they groom them and provide veterinary care, they work to rehabilitate those with behavioral problems, and they train volunteers who play with and exercise the animals each day. Humane societies often run programs in humane education, reaching out to groups ranging from school children to prison inmates. They may also offer obedience training classes, free or low-cost spaying and neutering services, pet food assistance for owners with limited incomes, and emergency relief during natural disasters. Wow. That is a tall order, but many humane societies do all of these things, and they do them well.

The lines that divide humane societies from municipal pounds may seem a little blurry. That's because they often work together and may even physically share the same space. In several communities that I have lived in, town governments paid for the housing and care of strays at the regional humane society. For a specific number of days, the owner could retrieve the lost pet, usually after paying a fine. If unclaimed, the animal became the responsibility of the humane society, where it usually was made available for adoption.

Because humane societies often serve more than one town, they usually have a fair number of dogs to consider for adoption (although they might not rival the number of animals in a big-city shelter). This gives you the advantage of a wide variety of dogs to consider. On any particular day, a dozen or more dogs may be available. And if you don't find the perfect pet, come back next week. There are sure to be others.

You should expect to pay a modest fee when you adopt a dog from a humane society. These organizations are usually not-for-profit. Aside from the salaries of key administrators, most of their funds go toward the animals. If you are asked to pay $60 for the adoption (as an example), you can safely assume that your new pet received many times that amount in food, grooming, and veterinary care, not to mention training and socialization efforts. Give more if you can. The compassionate and outstanding work of most humane societies truly deserves our support.

See Appendix B for a list of humane societies.

Other Nonprofit Groups

A separate category of adoption resources is the organizations that specialize in matching dogs and new owners. These groups typically do not have shelters themselves. Rather, they aid the work of humane societies and local pounds by connecting potential owners to adoptable dogs.

Some of these organizations are backed by individuals with big hearts and (often) big bank accounts. They may collect dogs from shelters, especially those animals that have "run out of time" and are close to being euthanized. Through networks of friends, celebrities, and business contacts, these groups recruit owners for these unwanted animals. They may showcase their animals in pet supply stores, in newspaper advertisements, or through newsletters. One group I've read about even has a "Petmobile," a large vehicle that brings adoptable dogs and cats to busy shopping centers in southern Florida.

Unlike humane societies, which often have a broad range of animal-

Adoptable Dogs on the Internet

What a concept! Adorable photos and appealing descriptions of thousands of adoptable dogs—all right at your fingertips. This is a resource that is still evolving. Internet adoption websites certainly expand an owner's options when he or she goes "dog shopping," but they will never, in my opinion, replace local adoption organizations. For pet owners, nose-to-nose contact is still the preferred way to size up a potential family member. By stroking, holding, and talking to a few dogs, owners get a sense of which dog feels right. And they also can get a sense of how the dog feels about them. These are important preliminaries to the bonding process. Imagine picking a dog from his mug shot in a canine lineup. It really is not an ideal way to get a dog.

On the other hand, the Internet is a great first step when browsing your local adoption organizations. Depending on the website's capabilities, you can check up on new arrivals, put yourself on a waiting list for a certain breed, view photos of the dogs, find a missing stray, and ask questions of the staff about one or more specific dogs. Internet contact will allow you to think through your adoption plans before you go to the shelter and are surrounded by all those needy animals. It can be a great asset in helping you to focus on choosing wisely and getting the right dog for you.

See Appendix A for some recommended websites.

related services, these nonprofits focus specifically on adoptions. Are they worthwhile? The ones I know about are outstanding. One of my favorites is Adopt-A-Dog, based in Greenwich, Connecticut. It serves the tristate area around New York City and has been matching people and dogs since 1981.

If you are not having success in finding a dog at your local pound or humane society, one of these adoption groups may be able to help you find the right animal. Exactly how do you find them? Check the Yellow Pages or speak to the staff at veterinary hospitals and boarding kennels. Local pounds and animal control officers may work directly with these groups and can put you in touch with them.

As with humane societies, be prepared to pay a fee or make a donation to support the organization's efforts. Although you may feel that you are doing *them* a service by adopting a dog, you should realize that they are really providing the service—of saving adoptable animals from death. I encourage you to support their efforts, which continue to be needed long after you take your own new pet home.

Breed Rescue Organizations

If you have strong feelings about owning a particular breed of dog, consider adopting one from a breed rescue group. These organizations, which may actually be solitary individuals doing Herculean work, are an outstanding resource for purebred dogs.

In my experience, many breed rescuers are dog breeders or long-time breed enthusiasts. They are knowledgeable about their breed and have a personal commitment to finding good homes for their charges. They are physically equipped to house several (sometimes many) dogs and can keep newcomers in separate runs until health and temperament are evaluated. Because they know their breed's behaviors, limitations, and common problems, they can screen the dogs for "adoptability" and even rehabilitate them when possible. They also know many owners who enjoy that breed and may be looking for another dog.

What kind of dog can you expect from a breed rescue organization? It's a mixed bag, ranging from new puppies (when a pregnant female is rescued) to canine senior citizens. Some are perfectly healthy; some

A Breed Rescuer's Tale

Adoption workers help a lot of dogs, and they end up with some great stories. One of my favorites is told by a longtime breeder and rescuer of Labrador retrievers, Julie Starkweather. Now semiretired, Julie has helped almost a thousand dogs find new homes. Winston was one of the memorable ones. Here's what she told me about him.

"I got a call from the local pound that there was a neutered black male Lab that was going to be destroyed. Of course, I went and got him. He was underweight and not neutered. He got all his shots, was wormed, neutered, etc., and back to my house he came.

"I always wait two weeks before trying to place a stray—to get to know them better—and oh, did I get to know this one. I named him Winston.

"Winston could clear my six-foot chain-link fence, and my invisible electric fence didn't faze him. He had to be from field lines and from a breeder, because his dewclaws had been removed. He liked playing with the other dogs, was smart and responsive, and would play fetch for hours. The minute he heard the kids next door he was over the fence, because he knew they would throw the ball for him. Needless to say, I knew this was not going to be an easy placement.

"Well, the dog god came through, and I received a call from the New York City Bomb Squad. They came and evaluated Winston. After they decided to take him, I warned them about his fence jumping. They told me not to worry as the kennel fencing was ten feet high and the rest of the area was sixteen feet. So off went Winston.

"The next day I got a call to tell me that Winston could not go over the sixteen-foot fence. But when they had arrived that morning, Winston was standing on top of the kennel building, having successfully scaled the ten-foot fence!

"Winston is now a five-year veteran of the bomb squad, and there are two other rescue dogs with him. Mayor Giuliani nicknamed him Winston the Wonder Dog."

I think that's short for "I wonder what amazing thing Winston will do next." Thank you, Winston, for your bravery and service. And thank you, Julie, for helping a death-row dog become a hero.

are middle-aged and sickly. The dogs may have turned up as random strays at the pound and been pulled in by the breed rescue group, or they may have been literally pulled off an urban street, as one breed rescuer I know did when she gave $10 to "a Brooklyn wino" for his tick-infested Lab, which successfully found a new home.

You can find breed rescue groups through veterinarians, regional kennel clubs, and breeders, and via the Internet on the American Kennel Club's website: www.akc.org/breeds/rescue. Do be prepared for a screening process when you express your interest in adoption. Breed rescuers are a devoted lot, and they have no interest in giving one of their beloved dogs to someone incapable of providing a good home. But if you qualify, lucky you. You will probably end up with a great dog, perhaps even a very valuable purebred dog, at minimal cost.

Greyhound Rescue

This breed rescue network deserves individual mention. Greyhounds are part of the "gaming" industry, that is, bets are placed on races in which these dogs compete. In short, racing greyhounds are bred for entertainment, and thousands of puppies are produced each year for this purpose. When the dogs are no longer winning, they are sometimes bred, often killed, and sometimes placed out for adoption.

Fortunately, the dog racing industry has become increasingly aware that many people abhor the killing of these animals. Track owners and kennel managers now often work together with adoption groups to find pet homes for some of their retired racers. Greyhound rescue groups can be found in many states, especially those with racing tracks. An Internet search or a phone call to a track can easily put you in contact with several organizations.

How are adopted greyhounds to live with? I don't have firsthand experience of living with one, but I have met many rescued "greys." They are amazing. I still remember my first meeting in the 1980s during an adult-education course I was teaching, called All About Dogs. A dog owner contacted me and asked to speak to my class on the relatively new subject of greyhound adoption. I cautiously agreed, because I expected to meet some uncontrolled, frenzied animals ready to run off at the slightest provocation. On the evening of my class, in walked two of the calmest, most obedient, most elegant, most graceful dogs I had ever seen. I was stunned.

Every adopted greyhound that I have met since then fits the same description. Owners tell me that they truly make wonderful pets and can live compatibly with other dogs, children, and even cats. Surprisingly, greyhounds have very modest exercise requirements, as they are sprinters, not long-distance runners. They are quite placid when indoors and are not at all yappy. Most racers are only a few years old when they are retired and made available for adoption. They live, on average, from twelve to fourteen years, giving their owners many years of companionship. I would put rescue greyhounds high on the list of great adoptable dogs.

Chapter 4

Picking the Perfect Pet

SO HOW DO YOU DECIDE? In some ways, this can be the toughest part of getting an adopted dog. If you visit a shelter, humane society, or rescue organization with many dogs needing homes, the screening process can be heartbreaking. A roomful of sad-eyed homeless dogs is enough to melt any animal lover's heart.

On the other hand, you may be offered a specific dog for adoption because of a particular situation. Your neighbors are moving and are giving up their pet, for example, or your adult son is off to graduate school. Aside from the pressure to accommodate your friends or relatives, these adoption decisions can be a bit easier, as you probably know the dog you're getting. This is a big advantage in your decision-making process. Still, you need to assess whether it is the right dog for you.

The Dog's Background

The more you know or can learn about an adoptable dog's background, the better. If you personally know the dog under consideration for adoption, you can assess, probably with good accuracy, its fit into your home. This dog may have visited with you, played in your backyard, slept over during a stint of pet-sitting, met your children or grandchildren, sniffed your cats, or cuddled in your lap. You have

Background Checklist

The more you know about a dog, the better prepared you are to make a good decision about adoption. You will also be better prepared to be a good owner. Use this checklist to determine what is known about your adoption candidate. It may be a lot or a little—depending on the dog's circumstances. Ask adoption workers, your veterinarian, or a professional trainer to help you assess some of the unknowns.

✳ Breed or mix of breeds
✳ Age
✳ Overall Physical condition
  Spayed or neutered?
  Previous pregnancies (for females)
  Coat and skin condition, including fleas or ticks
  Condition of teeth and gums
  Presence of cataracts in eyes
✳ Immunization history
✳ Temperament
  Interactions with strangers (you)
  Behavior in the shelter or pound
  Outgoing vs. shy
  Dominant vs. submissive
  Sensitivities to sound or objects
  A history of biting
✳ Previous home(s)
  Lived with dogs, cats, or other pets
  Lived with children (toddlers?)
  Lived with disabled family members
  A busy, multiperson household
    vs. a quiet home with a single owner
✳ Evidence of previous obedience training
✳ Evidence of previous abuse or neglect
✳ Reason the dog was given up for adoption

gained a good sense of the dog's personality, and the dog, in turn, has come to know you. If all seems well, go for it!

When you adopt a dog under such circumstances, there probably won't be too many unknowns. This is a good thing. You have a clear picture of the dog you are getting and are prepared to meet that dog's needs. In addition, the dog will be living with someone he knows. This can make his transition into a new home less stressful.

Unfortunately, this is an unlikely scenario. More often, you pick a cute face from among many homeless dogs at the local pound and hope for the best. But you can increase the odds of success by collecting as much information as possible about the dog.

Good humane societies and adoption organizations know that details about a dog's background help assure a successful adoption. When dogs are given up for adoption by their owners, shelter workers try to collect information about the dog's age, immunizations, health history, about interactions with other dogs, children, and cats, and about the reason(s) the dog is being given up. If the staff hears, "The dog bites my kids and fights with the neighborhood dogs," you can be sure that that animal will not be placed in a home with children and pets. In fact, an aggressive animal is unlikely to be placed in any home at all. Adoption workers are wise enough to avoid taking such risks.

Feedback from Experienced Handlers

Stray dogs and other dogs with unknown backgrounds can be the hardest to assess for adoption. No one has much information about them. Certainly a veterinarian can determine approximate age and general health as well as provide all current vaccinations. And shelter workers can share observations and opinions about the dog's temperament and behavior. But how is the dog to live with? It's hard to be sure.

One fortunate development in the world of adoption organizations is the increasingly widespread use of an on-site trainer. The trainer works with the adoptable dogs, often daily. Sometimes with the help of volunteers or a paid staff, the trainer puts the dogs through the paces of obedience training, meeting strangers, getting some exercise, interacting with other dogs, etc. Not only are the dogs learning a few useful skills, the shelter staff is getting to know the dogs.

I can't emphasize enough how valuable this information is. Put it to good use. If a shelter manager meets with you or collects information about you from an adoption application, he or she may have a strong sense that Little Dog A or Big Dog B is a good candidate for you. Consider this carefully. A professional who has interacted with hundreds or thousands of dogs has knowledge and an intuitive sense that most pet owners will never have. Unless the adoption worker strikes you as inexperienced, inattentive, or just plain out of touch (some are!), take his or her advice seriously.

Consulting a Veterinarian

A serious health issue or advanced age requires careful consideration. Sometimes the likelihood of healing or of a pain-free life is hard to estimate. In such cases, consult with a veterinarian about the dog you are considering. Learn whatever you can about the dog's condition. Veterinarians want homeless dogs to find homes, too. A responsible vet will give you the information you need to make a good decision.

A Dog's Appearance

Although much of this book is focused on behavior, it would be remiss to ignore the fact that a dog's appearance will influence your adoption choice. Owners are attracted to dogs of all colors, shapes, and sizes. Two dogs, side by side at the pound, might be fine adoption candidates for you. Appearance may be the only difference. For some reason, that scruffy face or that sleek coat or those bright eyes or that sad expression might touch a chord.

There's nothing wrong with this. Dog breeds were developed to satisfy human needs and whims. We humans have varied tastes, and fortunately, there are all kinds of dogs to suit them. Plus, I think it's important to like your dog's looks. The dog doesn't need to be purebred, show-quality perfect to be beautiful in your eyes. Your dog appeals to you simply for what he is.

Purebred vs. Mixed Breed

Some dog owners feel that purebred dogs are intrinsically more valuable than mutts. They are not. Sure they cost more and are eligible to enter dog shows, but those are characteristics invented by humans. In my opinion, every mentally sound, nonaggressive dog has the potential to be someone's wonderful pet.

Strictly speaking, *all* of our domestic dogs are mixed breeds. Each breed was created by combining traits of different kinds of dogs. After a certain number of generations, a true breed emerged. But mate a golden retriever with a German shepherd and you are back to a mutt, even though both parents were pedigreed for twenty generations.

Aside from snob appeal (if that matters to you), the main advantage of buying a purebred young dog is predictability, which I discussed in Chapter 2. Yet the advantage of adopting a specific adult dog (especially if the dog's history is known) is also predictability. What you see is what you get! The dog's size, shape, coat, health, and personality are all right before your eyes. That's a terrific advantage in finding a good pet.

My advice is not to get too focused on the issue of purebred versus mixed breed when selecting your adopted dog. If you do have a strong desire to own a particular breed, get in touch with a breed rescue organization. It will have plenty of adoptable dogs of the breed you want.

Interacting with the Dog

If you are getting a dog from a well-managed adoption organization, all of the available dogs will have been screened by an experienced trainer, kennel manager, or veterinarian. It is up to them—not you—to find signs of illness, physical faults, and serious behavior problems. In theory, any dog that you are allowed to see must meet certain minimum standards of sound health and temperament.

This means that you can pay more attention to things like personality and appearance. Keep in mind some of the basic criteria that you decided on in Chapter 2, "What Are You Looking For?" Your brain is

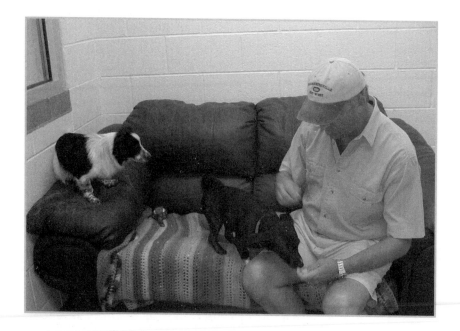

First impressions are important. Sit down to appear less threatening. Holding a small treat helps, too.

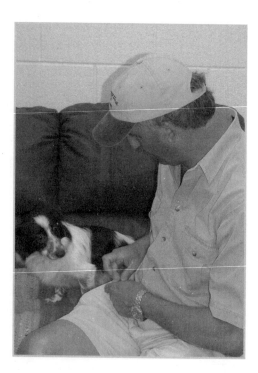

This nervous little dog is wary of the stranger but curious about the treat.

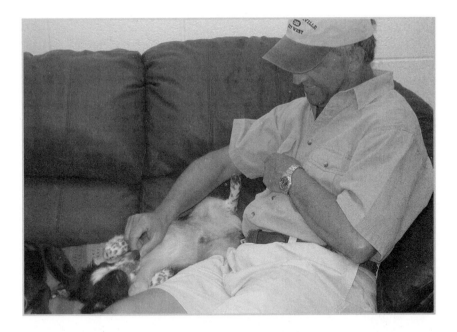

A "belly up" posture demonstrates a dog's submissive personality. If this dog were overly shy or frightened, he would not be taking the treat.

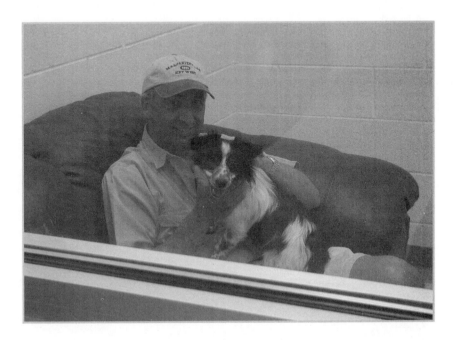

"I like this stranger now. Take me home!"

When You First Meet an Adoptable Dog

If an adoption worker does not give you specific directions for meeting and interacting with the dogs, follow these tips. They will help you—and the dog—make a good first impression.

✳ Relax. Act calmly and speak gently while meeting the dog.

✳ Sit on a chair to avoid seeming too dominant.

✳ Avoid direct eye contact at first, which can seem threatening to a dog.

✳ Reach out your hand, palm down, for the dog to sniff.

✳ Talk to the dog! Take note if your friendly words and demeanor get the dog's attention and get his tail wagging.

✳ Unless advised not to, pet the dog, rubbing behind his ears and scratching his chest or back.

✳ If the dog seems relaxed and interested in you, continue to handle him. You can try lifting a small dog into your lap or gently pressing a big dog's rump into a sit. Lift his lips to look at his gums. Take a paw and gently handle the foot. Continue talking to the dog as you do so.

✳ If the dog is wary or shy, do not force the handling issue. You do not want to frighten a nervous dog or provoke an aggressive one. Always use caution if you are not sure what to do.

✳ Have a few dog treats in your pocket. Unless you are told that the dog is on a special diet, give him a treat or two. Food almost always helps a stranger make a good first impression on a dog.

✳ If a fenced run is available, take the dog outside. Throw a ball or just walk around the enclosure together.

✳ Unless advised not to, clip a leash to the dog's collar and walk around for a few minutes.

✳ Look over your checklist regarding the dog's background.

✳ If the dog measures up, adopt him!

an important part of the decision-making process, but now is the time to listen to your heart, too.

When you meet one or more dogs, be prepared to follow the directions of the adoption worker. He or she may require that you adhere to a specific protocol when interacting with the dogs. This will be for your own safety and enjoyment as well as the comfort of the dogs and the liability of the shelter.

Meeting Adoption Candidates

I can offer a few general tips. Start with a calm and gentle demeanor. You want to make a positive first impression. A little exuberance is fine

Naming—or Renaming—Your Adopted Dog

Does it matter what you name your newly adopted dog? And do you have to stick with the name he came with, if you know it?

Dogs are adaptable creatures. You can feel free to choose a new name for your adopted dog if you like. After all, you are giving him a new life—one where he won't roam and where he will get nutritious food and regular health care, appropriate training, and lots of love. These may be much bigger changes for your dog than the name he once knew!

It's also possible that an old name has lots of unpleasant associations for an abused or neglected dog. You may not know what those associations are, of course. A new name is actually an excellent idea for a dog of this sort. It will be one of many signs that a better, happier life has just begun.

Be sure to make only positive associations with your adopted dog's name. A common mistake is to correct a dog by yelling his name. Your dog's name should never be used in this way. It will only teach the dog to ignore you when you use his name appropriately—to get his attention or call him to you. Chapter 6, "Canine Communication," gives more information on effective ways to speak to your dog.

for a boisterous dog, but a stranger may easily frighten a shy or inse-
cure dog. If possible, sit on a chair to reduce your imposing presence.
Body language is important to dogs (see Chapter 6), so use it to convey a friendly, inviting feeling.

Rather than reaching out and grabbing the dog, let him sniff your
outstretched hand and approach you. This may take a few minutes, or
he may jump right into your lap! These are the kinds of clues that will
give you a sense of the dog's personality and his feelings toward you.

Unless the adoption counselor advises against it, stroke the dog's
back, rub his ears, and scratch his chest. Don't be afraid to talk to the
dog, either. Does he respond in a positive way? Do you like what you
see? Try to get a sense of how you feel toward the dog as you interact.

I cannot tell you exactly how you'll know which dog you will want.
Something will speak to your heart or mind, and the fit will seem
right. Or maybe no dog will seem like a good match on that particular day. Try again next week or at a different shelter or adoption organization. There are a lot of dogs out there.

Yours at Last

When you have selected the right dog for you, the adoption counselor
may have additional questions, require additional paperwork, or
describe the next steps in an adoption protocol. Or maybe you will
just clip a leash to the dog's collar, and you and your adoptee can walk
out the door together. Happy day!

Whatever the timetable, be prepared at home with dog food and a
food bowl, a water bowl, a bed or crate, and a lot of time and attention for your new family member. A smooth start will make a big difference. Part Two will show you how.

Part Two

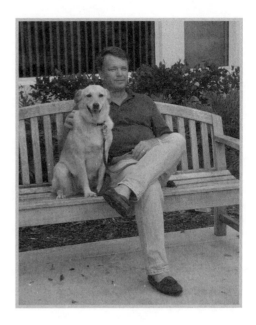

Off to a Good Start

Your adopted dog may have slept in more places than George Washington. Providing security, structure, and a sense of permanence is now your responsibility. So is helping to build trust. Here's how.

Chapter 5

A Dog-Friendly House and Yard

ONE OF THE BEST WAYS to help your adoption get off to a good, even a great, start is to turn your home into a dog-friendly place. What does this mean? In general, it means that your household routines, priorities, and physical space (indoors and out) will joyfully accommodate a dog.

This means different things for different households. Will your adopted dog have the run of the house or stay in a few designated rooms? How will you keep him out of the toddler's play area? Where will the dog sleep? Will you need to fence your yard? Stop home every lunch hour to let your dog out? These sorts of questions point out the realities of dog ownership. By opening your heart and home to an adopted dog, you have to be prepared with a dog-friendly environment. This chapter will help you do that.

Family Dynamics

The dynamics of most families work fine when an adopted dog joins the household. The presence of very young or very old family members may require you to be prepared in a special way.

Young children

A family with a newly adopted dog and a new baby needs to be ready for a lot of work. Any parent knows why. Babies require a lot of atten-

Dog Care Basics

Your dog-friendly house should be prepared with basic dog-care supplies, even before your adopted dog arrives home. Look over this list to make sure you have everything you need.

✳ *Food bowl and food.* If possible, continue feeding the same food that your adopted dog was previously eating. You can gradually switch him over to whatever food your veterinarian recommends. Also follow your veterinarian's advice on how much and how frequently to feed. Most dogs are fed once or twice a day.

✳ *A separate water bowl.* Your dog should always have access to clean water. Change the water every day, and wash the bowl once a week (or more) to prevent bacteria growth.

✳ *Leash and collar.* Lots of information on these essentials can be found in Chapter 18, "Using the Right Equipment."

✳ *Comb and brush.* Even if you will take your dog to a professional groomer, keep these supplies on hand. Many dogs enjoy the attention of frequent brushings, plus it allows you to check your dog for cuts or scrapes, ticks, fleas, suspicious lumps, or anything else that needs medical attention.

✳ *Toenail clippers.* See Chapter 28, "Grooming Tips," for a description of how to use these. Or ask your veterinarian or groomer to show you how. Check your dog's nails once a week, and trim as needed.

✳ *Dog towels.* This is what I call my big stack of old bath towels. I use them for drying wet dogs, cleaning up accidents or spills, covering a car seat for the dog, providing a temporary bed, etc. When you accumulate too many, drop some off at your local animal shelter. They use them, too.

✳ *A kennel crate,* if you will be using one for housebreaking. See Chapter 9.

✳ *A dog bed,* preferably in your bedroom to avoid isolating the

(continued)

dog at night. (See Chapter 8, "Bonding from Day One.") You may want to have additional dog beds in the family room, kitchen, dog room, etc.—wherever your dog will "hang out" and need a place to be comfortable. Your own furniture is fine, of course, but dog beds are a lot easier to clean.

tion and family adjustment. The same often holds true for households with toddlers and preschoolers. The supervision that these youngsters need can make it difficult to focus on a new dog.

You can help an adopted dog feel he belongs to your child-focused household by setting aside time each day just for him. Play ball for a while, practice obedience exercises, brush his coat—or all three. Give him the predictability of daily attention from you, even if it is brief at times. Also, include the dog with your children when you can. Practice Down-Stay while you read to the kids or feed the baby. Take a leash *and* stroller walk, so you all get some fresh air together. The more opportunities you find for safe and supervised time with both dog and child, the sooner your adopted dog will bond with your child and learn to behave properly in his or her presence. Chapter 29, "Kids and Dogs: Play It Safe," provides additional tips for success.

Baby gates are one of the best investments you can make for a household with dogs and young children. When my own family had one toddler and four dogs, we owned five baby gates. I called them "crowd control." We could keep the dogs downstairs or in the mudroom or out of the kitchen, depending on what we were doing and where our toddler was playing. Of course, the dogs often interacted with our child, but baby gates gave us the ability to control when and where that happened.

Seniors

At the other end of the human lifespan are elderly concerns. Households with seniors can be great dog-owning families. An elderly grandparent living in the home of younger family members can be a wonderful asset in an adopted dog's life. I've known families where the resident senior was the dog's special chum, providing daily brushings, neighborhood walks, and steady companionship while the rest of the family rushed around in their busy lives.

There is also the possibility that an elderly family member will be vastly unhappy about an adopted dog's arrival. In generations past, it was more common for a family dog to live in the backyard or the barn—not in the house. Seeing Poopsie Poodle curled up on the bed or licking up crumbs in the kitchen could make Grandpa's blood boil. A dog that gets into things, such as Grandma's knitting or her medications, is indeed a nuisance and an unfair disruption to her routine. And any dog that jumps on or bumps into people is an actual danger to a frail senior who is no longer steady on his or her feet.

Crowd control, with baby gates, closed doors, and supervision, is your best tool for helping an adopted dog and an elderly family member enjoy living together. Obedience training will also make a big difference. A dog that can lie down and stay, walk calmly on a leash, and greet people without jumping is a dog that can interact safely with most seniors. Put these exercises at the top of your training list, especially if your adopted dog is big and energetic. It will speed up the dog's welcome into your elderly family member's heart.

Work schedules

Working is part of life, and for the most part, people work outside their homes. How does this fit in with responsible dog ownership? For one thing, it means that if your house is empty ten to twelve hours a day on a regular basis, you really have no business owning a dog. Dogs are social animals. Asking a dog to live essentially alone is not doing the dog any favors. Get an aquarium if you want to come home to pets after a long day at the office. If you imagine a big, wagging dog greeting you calmly at the door after twelve hours alone, keep that vision in your imagination and enjoy it there. It has no place in the reality of dog ownership.

Yet lots of working people are good dog owners. How? Perhaps they have a spouse or roommate at home. Or they work reasonably short hours and/or come home for lunch each day. Maybe they pay a pet sitter to stop in midday to exercise the dog and give him a bathroom break. Perhaps they own several dogs so that the dogs have companionship. Some people can even bring their dogs to work.

These scenarios give you some idea of how your working life can mesh with your dog-owning life. Remember that adopting a dog means giving the dog a home, not just a house to live in. Your presence is an important part of the picture.

Allergy management

Sad but true: Some unfortunate people are allergic to dogs. This is occasionally the reason that healthy, well-trained, wonderful dogs are given up for adoption. My brother-in-law's family came to own a sweet, middle-aged poodle because of allergies. Tootsie was a great pet and even enjoyed short visits with her first family, but their child's severe allergies prevented Tootsie from living with them full time.

If you are the one with dog allergies, consider adopting one of the breeds that tend to cause fewer allergy problems. Schnauzers, poodles, and some terriers make this list. Keep the dog off your bed or out of the bedroom altogether. As frequently as possible, wash the dog beds, vacuum the house, and have a groomer bathe the dog. Wash your hands after brushing or cuddling your dog.

These measures might not be enough. You may need medical intervention to live compatibly with your adopted dog. Seek out the care of an allergist to learn about additional household changes, medications, and therapies that can help.

House Size and Style

Will your adopted dog fit your home? Size does matter in making your house a dog-friendly home. A Great Dane in an antique-filled studio apartment cannot move without mishap in such a confined space. Common sense will tell you if the physical traits of your home are appropriate for your adopted dog. There should be room enough for the dog to walk around, relax, and sleep comfortably without crashing into things or disrupting other family members. If the whole house or apartment will not be open to the dog, there should be plenty of dog-friendly areas. After all, you are getting a dog to live with *you*, not with your walls, doors, and furniture.

Decorating styles are irrelevant to dogs, but they matter to some dog-owning humans. Is your house style dog-friendly? If your entire palace is done in ivory, a Labrador retriever may shed too much black fur for your pleasure. White terriers can do a number on navy or brown upholstery.

Am I suggesting that you color-coordinate your dog with your house? Or vice versa? It's been done, of course. In fact, I've even seen books and articles on the subject. More realistically, just make sure that your home is reasonably capable of housing an animal. During the course of their lifetimes, dogs may vomit, suffer from diarrhea, lose bladder control because of illness or old age, bleed from a wound, ooze from an infection, drip mud after a walk, shake off water after a bath, and shed fur. You wouldn't kick a human member out of your family for these behaviors, so don't do it to a dog, either. Be prepared for a little mess.

A Dog Room

One way that many owners successfully manage dog ownership—and deal with occasional messiness—is to have a "dog room." This can be a laundry room, mudroom, bathroom, entryway, stair landing, etc. Generally speaking, it is a space that opens into a living area (to avoid isolating the dog) but can be blocked off with a baby gate (preferably) or closed door (if necessary). The dog room is where the dog dries off after a bath or a rainy-day walk. It is where he spends the day during a bout of diarrhea. Food and water bowls are here, keeping crumbs and splashes somewhat confined. A dog bed or kennel crate provides a comfortable place to sleep if this is where the dog hangs out when you leave the house. A nearby cupboard can hold dog food, grooming supplies, leash and collar, and a stack of old towels for drying off and cleaning up.

The layout of your home will somewhat determine if you can create a dog room. Some owners designate their bedroom or family room as the dog room, making sure that floor coverings and furniture can be easily cleaned when necessary. I've also met owners whose whole

Dog-Proofing Your Home and Yard

Most people know about baby-proofing a home so that a curious tod-dler cannot be easily harmed. You can dog-proof your home and yard, too, to help keep your adopted dog safe in his new environment.

All of these suggestions may not apply to your specific home. Other steps may also be needed that are not mentioned here. The size, strength, and age of your adopted dog will somewhat deter-mine your dog-proofing needs. But if in doubt, do it. Your dog's safety may depend on it one day.

* Secure electrical cords, especially from table lamps. A dan-gling cord can be pulled or entangled by a dog, dragging a heavy lamp or an appliance onto the floor.
* Put your kitchen trash can in a pantry or cupboard. Or buy one with a lid. Chicken bones and other garbage should not be part of your dog's diet.
* Put candy dishes on high shelves, not low tables. Chocolate in particular is toxic to dogs.
* Check the security of windows and window screens. You don't want a little dog falling out or a big dog pushing through.
* Cover electrical outlets with plastic safety caps if your dog shows any interest in licking or sniffing them. Spray electrical cords with Bitter Apple (or similar product) to discourage chewing on them.
* Check your fenced yard for escape routes. Repair or block them up.
* Ask a landscaper or experienced gardener to look over your shrubbery, flowerbeds, and houseplants for plant dangers.
* Clean up spills or drips from automobiles in the garage or driveway. Most antifreeze tastes sweet to dogs, but it is highly poisonous.
* Cover your backyard pool or fence it off to restrict the dog's access. Dogs really do get into pools and drown, even during cold weather.   *(continued)*

Dog-Proofing Your Home and Yard *(continued)*

* Provide for safe travel in your vehicle. This may mean purchasing a travel crate, a seat-belt restraint harness, or a behind-the-seat gate to secure the dog in the back. Safe travel does *not* mean letting the dog ride loose in an open pickup truck. This is now illegal in many locations because so many dogs have been killed or injured as a result.

* Decide on a sanitary plan for disposing of feces. In my backyard I keep a lidded trashcan lined with a large plastic bag for this purpose. After I scoop up after my dog, the waste goes in there and can later be discarded. City dwellers will need to have a supply of small bags for cleaning up sidewalks and curbs.

house is a dog room! As long as you don't mind cleaning up a lot, do whatever works for you. But from experience, I can assure you that a specific space will help make dog ownership a bit easier.

A Place to Eliminate

A dog's need to eliminate must be accommodated in a sanitary way. A little Yorkie living on the forty-fourth floor of a Manhattan high-rise can probably urinate and defecate on newspapers for his entire lifetime without causing too much odor or mess (as long as there is frequent cleanup). But don't expect a mastiff to live like that.

The great outdoors is where most people take their dogs to eliminate. Think through a realistic plan as you contemplate dog adoption. Will you leash-walk your dog several times a day? Perhaps you have a fenced yard where the dog can run around and eliminate. A nearby park might work, but remember that early-morning and late-night outings will be required every day in every kind of weather. Don't make your plans too impractical, or you and your dog will both be miserable.

I have found that a grassy or sandy area close to the house works great. It's convenient for humans and dogs alike. Urban dog owners might be challenged to find someplace like this. If so, plan to invest in scooper bags for sidewalk cleanup. There is no excuse for leaving your dog's excrement where it can offend others. Even backyards need to be cleaned frequently. Chapter 9, on housebreaking, will help you teach your dog to go there reliably.

Preventing Roaming

Dogs, by nature, are wanderers. Open the back door, and nine times out of ten a dog will wander off to see the world—or at least the neighborhood. Your adopted dog is no different. In fact, his urge to roam may be especially strong if he was once a chronic wanderer or homeless street waif.

Your job is to keep your adopted dog safe at home in your house or yard. This might not be as easy as it sounds. I remember one client whose dog was always getting out of the house. Her four children were in and out all day, and a poorly latched door was easy for the dog to push open. My advice to her was to "tighten the ship." This meant repairing the door latch and teaching the kids to close the door securely. It also meant paying closer attention to the dog and kids, keeping their whereabouts on her mind.

A few decades ago, it was common practice to open the back door and let the dog out. He came back when he was good and ready. *Times have changed.* Leash laws in most communities impose stiff fines on owners with loose dogs. And the risks to a wandering dog are great. Traffic accidents, dogfights, poisons, wild animals, and even dognapping can await an unsupervised, roaming dog. If your dog ends up lost and in a distant pound, he may not get a new owner as caring as you. In fact, he might not get a new owner at all. Euthanasia is a likely fate.

A fenced yard

If your home has a yard, secure fencing is the best way to keep your dog in while still allowing him to play freely outdoors. A variety of materials work fine: chain link, metal railing, wooden boards, even

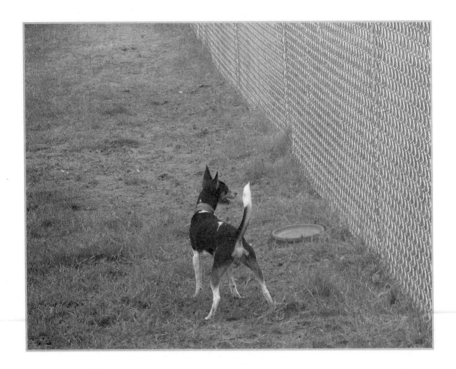

A dog-friendly yard is one that keeps a dog from roaming. Fencing is one of the best investments you can make in your adopted dog's safety.

inexpensive garden wire mesh mounted to metal stakes. Your budget and community regulations may dictate which you choose. So will the size, strength, and jumping ability of your dog.

Invisible "pet containment systems" also work well. These consist of a buried wire around the yard's perimeter and a transmitter collar worn by the dog. When the dog approaches the wire, he hears a warning beep. If he continues across, he receives an electric shock correction. A specific training program teaches the dog to back up into the yard instead of running across to freedom. These systems are useful in areas where traditional fencing is prohibited or unsightly.

An advantage of invisible fencing is that you can create a dog-friendly area of almost any shape in any part of your yard. The underground wire, which rests just a few inches below the surface, can curve around flowerbeds, run along the pool deck, or block off the kids' swing set and sandbox. The dog can go outside without digging up tulips, jumping into the pool, or urinating where the kids play. Some of these systems are even modified for indoor use if certain rooms or furniture must be made off-limits.

A disadvantage to invisible fencing is that while it keeps your dog in the yard, it doesn't keep other dogs or wildlife out. Depending on your surrounding environment, this may or may not be a problem. Speak to local distributors or installers about specific concerns you might have. Neighbors may also be able to give you feedback if they are using this type of fencing.

Routines and Predictability

When you have created a dog-friendly house and yard with the help of this chapter, stick with what you have done for at least a few weeks before experimenting with additional changes. Your newly adopted dog will probably get used to your home before you know it, and you won't need to change a thing.

It's important to remember that many adopted dogs have spent weeks or months (or even years) living a tumultuous, stressful, and unpredictable life. A dog-friendly home with predictable household routines has a powerful effect on these dogs. They settle down. In such an environment, they are cared for, they are included in family life, and they know what to expect from one day to the next. That in itself will speed up your adopted dog's adjustment to his new life with you.

Chapter 6

Canine Communication

DOGS ARE NOT BORN understanding human language. They have a lot of exceptional abilities, but language is not one of them. Fortunately, they can learn to associate human words or phrases with specific behavior. These are words that have been spoken repeatedly to the dog, usually with a predictable result. For example, many owners would claim that their dog understands the phrase "Do you want to go out?" The dog, of course, can't answer with human language: "Sure, that sounds like a good idea." But their animated movements, running toward the door, barking, or jumping up, tell us that they know exactly what the owner has asked.

Obedience-trained dogs have been taught to respond in a specific way when they hear spoken words such as "sit," "down," or "come." And some dogs can learn to recognize the meaning of many words, even words strung together in a variety of ways. Drifter, my late, great Australian shepherd, would accurately obey this phrase: "Get your ball, and go lie down on your nest."

Yet dogs' ability to recognize human language is only part of their repertoire of communication skills. Dogs definitely have their own language, which is purely canine. Our ability to understand *their* language—and to put it to practical use—is important for a positive dog-human relationship. In my experience, obedience training is far easier and more effective when using canine language. And understanding this language is absolutely essential to any owner trying to sort through a dog's behavioral problems.

Dog Talk

Dogs rely a great deal on body language and scent to communicate with each other. This is where humans are at a disadvantage. For one, we don't have tails! Tails wag, point straight out, tuck under, etc. In certain situations we can "read our dogs" by interpreting what the tail is doing, but we can't reciprocate in the same way.

Body postures also convey meaning between dogs. Examples include the play-bow (front end lowered, hind end up in the air) and the various positionings of the ears. Plenty has been written about canine body postures, and excellent diagrams and interpretations can be found in several books. But humans can't really put this to extensive use. Rear ends and ears are not our most communicative assets. Fortunately, some simple movements, such as standing up, can be used. These are discussed later in this chapter.

Scent is hugely important for canine communication to a degree that we cannot even measure. Olfactory cues reveal where a dog has been, who it has met, what it has eaten, its current reproductive status, its age, its health, and probably dozens of other informational tidbits. It's likely that your dog knows these things about *you* from various scents on your person. In fact, a dog will recognize you by your scent alone. Each person's scent is an identifiable fingerprint, so to speak, but our own olfactory abilities cannot make use of this. You know next to nothing about your dog from olfactory clues.

I can think of just a few exceptions. We all know what creature a "skunked" dog recently met. And I know from my springer spaniel's breath when she has raided our cat's litter box. And stinky ears mean it's time to clean out the excess wax. But by and large, scent is not a way that humans and dogs can communicate very efficiently.

Which leaves us with sound. (Touch is important, too, especially for bonding with adopted dogs. It is discussed separately in Chapter 8.)

Dogs use sound—that is, verbal cues—for all sorts of purposes. They can produce a variety of whines, whimpers, barks, and growls, and they have excellent hearing for reception of these sounds.

Here are some examples. Dogs whine and bark a high-pitched yip when they are distressed from being separated or isolated from their pack. You may have heard your adopted dog whine and yip when she wanted to come in from outdoors or be let out of her crate. Mother dogs whimper to their puppies to call them to her.

Barking, the most familiar canine sound, has many different meanings. Dogs bark to alert the pack of an intruder or to drive the intruder away. They bark to stimulate and encourage play. They bark when startled or when they want attention. Byron, my spoiled black Lab, barked every afternoon when he wanted his dinner.

Growling is a warning sound. It is a dog's way of saying, "Stop what you are doing immediately!" A mother dog growls when her puppies nurse too vigorously or bite on her ears or legs. Puppies growl during play as they test their littermates to see who is the toughest. Dominant dogs growl at subordinates to warn them to stay away from their food or to back off and leave them alone. You may have observed this at the animal shelter if you saw several dogs interacting with one another.

Growling may escalate into an attack if the "growlee" does not respond to the warning. But fortunately, dogs know that. They learned it as puppies when mother dog snapped or bit when they did not heed her warning. In domestic dogs especially, respecting a growl is one of the most important lessons they learn in life. It makes them capable of responding to humans in the same way, which means, essentially, that they are capable of being trained and of living obediently with their human families.

After many years of working with dogs and their owners, I have come to the overwhelming conclusion that the best way to teach dogs is to communicate with them in their own language. Without the resources of a tail, movable ears, or high-level scent discrimination, humans can rely on something that *is* highly developed: their voice.

Vocal communication with dogs is not as far-fetched as it sounds. If you can growl and use a high-pitched praise tone, you can do it. Your adopted dog is not going to start speaking English or French to you, but you can start today speaking Canine to him. When you do, you will have a direct line into his brain, and you can use it to teach him all sorts of useful things.

Learning by Doing

Fortunately for us, dogs learn things in a fairly simple way. If they act and it is agreeable—that is, it feels good, smells good, sounds good, or tastes good—they will do it again. If a behavior results in something that is disagreeable—it feels bad, smells bad, sounds bad, or tastes bad—they will avoid doing it.

This is a bit simplistic, of course, because other factors come into play. The intensity of the response matters. For example, one burned nose from sniffing a hot woodstove may be all it takes to teach a dog to permanently avoid the woodstove.

The dog's personality matters, too. A dog that adores hunting and catching prey may continue to do so, even when a porcupine, for example, gives him an unpleasant quill attack. And timing of the dog's experience is significant as well. A dog that licks sweet-tasting automotive antifreeze won't associate the severe, life-threatening sickness he experiences hours later as a result of his action. That is because the sickness is not connected immediately in time with licking the toxin.

Most learning experiences do not happen quickly. Dogs typically learn most things by doing them many times over and over again until they have formed a habit. That's when we can say that our dogs "know" something.

Which brings us back to "agreeable" and "disagreeable." I correct dogs by creating a disagreeable response to any undesirable behavior. Basically, I growl at them. I learned this from dogs themselves. Puppies learn from their mothers that a growl means "Stop!" When I want to tell a dog to immediately stop whatever he is doing, I growl, imitating mother dog. With few exceptions, every dog that I have ever met knows what I mean.

What does my growl sound like?

My growl does not sound like "Grrrrr." This spelling reminds me of what a comic-strip artist might write next to a grizzly bear to represent growling. My growl is more canine—that is, guttural. Say "Nhaa!" as sharply and deeply in your throat as possible. When you can feel vibrations below your Adam's apple, you're growling.

But sounding exactly like me is not the goal. What is most important is your tone, not the specific word. The tone must be low and deep from the throat.

Many trainers believe that the most important obedience command a dog should learn is "No." I agree with this philosophy. A guttural "Nhaa!" is simply a variation of the word "No." They both mean to stop whatever you are doing immediately.

Keep in mind that it is not the word that the dog understands. It is all in the tone. "No, sweetie, please don't do that to Mommy's sofa," said in a soft, pleasant, high-pitched tone, will not communicate what you want. However, "No!" or "Nhaa!" delivered in a low, tough, guttural tone will be interpreted as a growl. *That* will stop your dog from chewing on the sofa.

Personally, I find "Nhaa!" to be even more effective as a growl than "No." "No" is a conversational word, while "Nhaa!" is distinctive-sounding and has one specific meaning.

No matter what word you use to mean "Stop," the sound must be guttural to be effective. It takes a little bit of practice to master a good "Nhaa!" but I have taught people from age five to eighty-five to growl. You must work on tone in order to effectively talk dog.

All dogs are different

You must vary your "Nhaa!" correction according to the personality and temperament of your dog. I have worked with extremely sensitive dogs that have required no more than a barely audible "Nhaa!" to get the message across. On the other hand, I have worked with individuals that I have had to, on occasion, growl at loud and long.

As a rule, intense volume is not necessary. Screaming, ranting, and raving at a dog are generally ineffective. Doing so will in all likelihood teach your dog to tune you out. Always start with a low, guttural "Nhaa!" If you must, bring the volume up a notch to make your point—but do not allow it to turn into a scream.

The invisible leash

One of the great things about a verbal correction is that once the dog has learned it, you will have excellent off-leash control of your dog. For example, if my springer spaniel, Crea, does not respond immediately to the Come command, just a quick "Nhaa!" will get her attention and a response. Now that she is eight years old, the amount of growling that I have to do is minimal. But it is still a sound that I can use anywhere, anytime, to stop whatever she is doing wrong.

Using Body Postures to Communicate with Your Dog

Although we don't have ears and tails to match our dogs, we can imitate one body posture quite effectively. That is a dominant stance over the dog. If your dog ignores your growl, enhance your growl's effectiveness with dominant body posture. This is better than bringing up the volume of your growl.

Here is an example. If your dog is starting to chew the rug while you are sitting on the sofa watching TV, you should growl "Nhaa!" If the dog stops chewing, great. That's the result you wanted. If he does not stop, you should get up and stand over him and growl. In all likelihood he will stop.

When I correct my dogs I use a lot of theatrics. When I growl, for example, I stand up and use that guttural tone along with facial expressions to convey that I am a tough pack leader. My goal is to swiftly and effectively communicate to my dog that I mean business. Keep mother dog in mind. She doesn't plead and whine and beg her pups to stop biting at her paws. She growls or even snaps, and it's over.

I never allow puppies or adult dogs to frustrate me into becoming angry or violent. Any time you react to a dog out of anger, it is a losing situation. My verbal tone and body language are all an imitative display designed to communicate with the dog in his language.

Bad Training Methods

For too many years, dog trainers have used heavy-handed and sometimes outright abusive training methods. When I first started training dogs in 1972, methods such as kneeing dogs in the chest to teach them not to jump on people were commonplace. In some of the early training classes that I attended, obedience instructors would "string up" dogs that were excited and became overly stimulated by the distractions of a group class. The dog's only "crime" was having a hard time sitting and staying.

To string up a dog means to literally hang a dog by pulling up on the leash, lifting the dog's front legs off the ground. Doing this causes the choke collar to constrict around the dog's throat, cutting off his breathing. I've seen trainers do this to dogs for thirty seconds or more until the dog was on the fringe of blacking out. Needless to say, it would have a calming effect on the dog. It also taught the dog something—to fear the trainer and often its owner. It also taught the dog to hate obedience training. This "technique" is dog abuse and should be against the law. I no longer attend other instructors' training classes and do not know if this still goes on. It is an example of a bad, abusive, and completely inappropriate way to correct a dog's behavior.

Praising Your Dog

Life with a dog is not all growling and corrections. On the contrary! Praise is an integral part of communicating with your dog. A well-trained dog knows the household rules, knows how to behave outdoors, has self-control when walking on a leash, and minds his manners around family members and strangers. This is the kind of dog we all strive for, and it is a dog that is praised and rewarded daily for being so wonderful.

Let's evaluate different kinds of praise and rewards from a canine point of view. Nothing is better for most dogs than food. Dog treats, table scraps, and even the daily bowl of kibble are high points in the day for most dogs. This makes food a desirable reward for good behavior.

Crea, my springer spaniel, has a favorite morning chore: She fetches the newspaper from the end of the driveway. She loves to step outside to get the early-morning smells. She also loves to fetch and carry things. And she is happy and proud of herself when we tell her, "Good girl, Crea!" But she *really* loves the dog biscuit that is part of her reward for bringing in the news.

This brings us to verbal communication again. Dogs respond in a positive way to high-pitched voices. Mother dog called to her pups with a squeaky-sounding whimper, and they happily came running to her. My all-time favorite experience with this behavior took place when I met a litter of six-week-old wolf puppies at a sanctuary in Connecticut. The mother wolf was not with them, and they acted extremely shy and nervous of the newcomer (me). Always thinking like a dog, I lay on the floor on my back and did my best imitation of a mother dog's whimper. Six baby wolves came running over. They sniffed and licked me all over the face! It was intensely wonderful.

That experience reinforced a few things in my understanding of canines. High-pitched sounds are reassuring and pleasing to a dog. A nonthreatening body posture is equally important. Emulating canine vocal tones and body language are the keys to canine communication. And puppy breath—even in wolves—smells sweet.

So praise your dog with a high-pitched, affectionate voice. "Good dog! What a good girl you are!" is sure to get your dog's tail wagging with happiness. Couple that with a gentle petting or shoulder rub, and you have indeed found a way to praise and reward your dog in her own language.

Ready to Take Charge

One of the most important first steps in your relationship with your adopted dog is establishing yourself as the pack leader. Turning your adopted dog into an obedient, well-behaved member of your family depends on it. With your vocal cords warmed up and a basic understanding of canine body language, you are prepared to take charge. The next chapter will show you how.

Chapter 7

Taking Charge: What It Means to Be Pack Leader

DOGS AND HUMANS have a unique relationship, because dogs view humans in a way that no other domestic animals do.

Cats coexist with us. They let us feed them. When they are in the right mood, they let us pet and handle them. Still, I don't believe they feel they are human. And they *know* we are not cats. In fact, cats would probably be insulted at the thought of being human!

Horses let us ride them. They nibble carrots and apples from our hands. But they don't think they are the same as us. Try thinking about other kinds of pets—goldfish, parrots, hamsters, rats, guinea pigs. None of these animals relate to humans the way dogs do. Only dogs view humans as though we are both one and the same.

Look at the many similarities between us. Canines are social animals that live together in packs. Humans live together in families and communities. Individuals of both species have specific roles and functions within the group. Both perform behaviors such as hunting, guarding, and rearing young in order to enhance the overall good of the group. Human societies have a hierarchy system of leaders and followers, which helps us to maintain order and harmony. This is true in a canine pack as well.

Domestic dogs—when they are cared for and treated well—view our families as their packs. They help to protect our property and us. How many countless stories have been told of the family dog saving one of the children? Dogs sleep with us and hunt with us. They work with humans in the police and military forces as valued and devoted partners. They lead the blind and assist people with physical challenges. They cheer sick and elderly people with their visits. I do not believe that all of this would be possible if dogs did not feel that they were only doing what is natural to them—sharing in the lives of their family members.

Your adopted dog is a pack animal that must adjust to living with his new pack (you and your family). You can help his adjustment tremendously by being a good pack leader. Consider first how puppies develop their pack skills, described below. If you understand this important component of canine behavior, you can establish a healthy, orderly pack environment in your own home. Getting off to a good start with your adopted dog depends on it.

Learning How to Live in a Pack

Even before they join a human family, most dogs start off in the world with a pack and a pack leader. Littermate brothers and sisters and mother dog fulfill this role. They provide puppies with an invaluable learning experience: how to be a pack animal.

At about three weeks of age, puppies' ears and eyes open. The youngsters start to learn the techniques that are required to function in a pack. They learn when to be tough and assertive and when to be submissive and to follow direction. For example, puppies will compete with each other for food. They will snap and growl at each other. They will climb on, bark at, and bite each other.

With each passing day and week, the pecking order of the puppy pack takes shape. A dominant puppy will emerge. This individual will eat the most, bark the loudest, and growl the fiercest. He or she will bully the other littermates around.

I once asked an experienced Labrador retriever breeder which gender usually became the dominant puppy in a litter. She replied, "Either the biggest male or the female with the biggest mouth." That's a testimony to the significance of a good, tough growl.

Sometimes the pecking order among the puppies is very obvious. Other times it is not so clear. Experienced breeders usually know. By the time a litter of puppies is eight weeks old, they can often point out which of the puppies is the most dominant and which is the most submissive. The puppies are learning to be pack animals.

Mom rules

Fortunately, mother dog usually asserts herself within the litter as the undisputed pack leader. A good mother dog disciplines even the most dominant puppy in the litter. For example, when a puppy nurses too vigorously or chews on Mom's legs or ears, she will correct the pup. This motherly discipline teaches all puppies how to act submissively and reverently toward a leader.

Mother dog primarily corrects her puppies by growling at them. When she wants to tell a puppy, "Stop it," she says it with a firm, guttural growl. If the puppy ignores her growl she may escalate her aggression by snapping at him. I have even seen a mother dog nip a puppy and cause him to yip.

I have seen mother dogs raise their lip and growl at their seven- and eight-week-old puppies from about three feet away. In the beginning of my career, I remember being confused by this behavior. I asked the breeder, "Why is she doing that? Doesn't she like her pups?" The breeder replied, "Oh, she likes her pups perfectly well. She just knows that they are thinking about pouncing on her or nipping her leg. She is just telling them, 'Don't even think about it.'" That's an astute parent! The timing of her correction prevented the puppy from even *starting* an unwanted behavior.

Cousin Wolf

In the wolf pack there is an alpha male and alpha female that dominate the pack. Unlike domestic canine "puppy packs," wolves live in packs that include extended family. The father, aunts, uncles, and cousins from previous litters make up the typical wolf pack. It is probable that if a domestic dog pack became feral (semiwild), it would change over time to resemble the structure of a wolf pack.

Left intact, a puppy pack would also evolve over time as the puppies matured. Changes in pack ranking would probably occur. However, this process is interrupted when puppies are sold or given away, generally at around eight weeks old. Puppies are separated from their pack and join a new pack: their human family.

Take me to your leader

The biggest misconception about dogs is that they want to please all humans. This is not true. Dogs only want to please their pack leader. If a human is viewed by a dog as pack leader, the dog will want to please that person. This is the foundation for dog obedience training.

Your adopted dog must develop the willingness to please you if you expect the dog to respond reliably to your commands. Dogs that view themselves as the pack leader will never be obedient to their owners. They will naturally expect fellow pack members to want to please them.

Every dog, no matter what its age, will be attuned to pack dynamics in its new human family. This goes for eight-week-old puppies as well as adolescent and older dogs. Your adopted dog is no different. He will seek a place in his pack where he best fits in.

This may happen without any disruption or even visible effort. Or it may be a tumultuous struggle that eventually makes your adoption effort a failure. Described here are factors that affect how well—or how poorly—your adopted dog settles into the pack hierarchy of your household. Included are tips for being a good pack leader and inspiring harmony within your pack.

Helping Your Adopted Dog Fit In

Every responsible owner of an adopted dog wants to help the new pet adjust quickly and peacefully into his new home. By being a good pack leader, you can greatly influence how well that happens. But there are some factors that you cannot control. They come with the dog. Fortunately, you can make an effort to understand these factors and to respond appropriately. The peace in your pack depends on it.

Youth

As described above, puppies are learning about pack hierarchy. By playing, wrestling, competing for food, mouthing, biting, growling, etc., they are testing their own feelings of dominance and submission. It is natural and appropriate for them to have these behaviors. Unfortunately, these behaviors are not so appropriate in a human pack. Owners do not want a big, goofy seven-month-old dog mouthing their arms, knocking over their children, or snapping at anyone near the food dish.

If you have adopted a puppy or adolescent dog, be prepared to deal with these behaviors. How you respond to them is extremely important if you want the dog to grow into a sweet, well-behaved adult. Essentially, you must become the pack leader in your dog's eyes.

Your dog's breed

I hate to generalize. Like humans, dogs are individuals that have unique, interesting personalities. However, human intervention into dog breeding has produced specific breeds with distinct characteristics. Collies have long coats; poodles have curly coats. Rottweilers are big; Chihuahuas are small.

To succeed at the jobs they were bred to do, dogs also have breed-specific personality traits. These are not as cut-and-dried or as predictable as the size of a Chihuahua or the curly coat of a poodle, but general personality trends clearly exist in all breeds. This may affect your dog's pack mentality and its willingness to accept you as pack leader.

Consider these examples. Sled dogs tend to be stubborn. Terriers excitable. Labs and goldens friendly. Guard dogs wary and aggressive. Your adopted dog may not have the "typical" personality for his breed (or mix of breeds), but it is probable that he will have some predictable tendencies. These may influence the challenges you face in establishing yourself as pack leader. Consider what your dog was bred to do, and also gather information and advice from breed books and experienced breeders. They will help you better understand your dog.

A dominant personality

Most truly dominant dogs were born that way. Their breed, size, and current age are irrelevant. Occasionally, dogs with only moderate innate dominance have had life experiences that built their confidence and strengthened their dominant attitudes. But most dominant dogs are naturally, in their hearts, down to their toenails born to be in charge.

These can be tough dogs to live with. They are not inclined to obey anyone. They may growl at or rough up other dogs in the household. They may growl at family members and may not tolerate children. They may be too aggressive in guarding the house or yard, even from friends or neighbors.

Dominant dogs need owners with a strong pack-leader image. These dogs need clear rules of acceptable and unacceptable behavior—even though they may test those rules every day or week of their lives. They also need consistency. With some dominant dogs, any bending of the rules into "maybe" or "sometimes" only communicates that no one is really in charge. It is a signal to the dog that now is his chance to take over the pack. Aggression and other threatening behaviors can start to appear.

Owners never need to hit, kick, or be abusive to manage a dominant dog. All they need to do is think and act—and respond to problems—as a pack leader would. It all goes back to my philosophy of training dogs through a canine point of view. Here's how.

The Pack Leader: You

As mentioned above, pack leaders have certain traits that allow them to maintain harmony and control in their packs. Consistency, good timing, and certain body language are the most important in the pet home. These traits come naturally to some owners. Others have to work at it.

Although extremely submissive dogs need gentle, nonthreatening handling, they too must understand that you are in charge (see Chapter 14). In contrast, some highly dominant dogs need an especially strong pack leader if they are going to live successfully in a human home. Most dogs fall somewhere in the middle of those extremes. Yet all must take direction from their owners—not the other way around.

Consistency with corrections

An important pack-leader trait is consistency. When a canine exhibits unwanted behavior (mouthing, food stealing, etc.), the pack leader responds with a correction *every time*. In a wolf pack this might mean a growl, a bite, a dominant stance, or even a fight.

In a human pack, an owner should growl "Nhaa!" This sound, given in a deep, guttural tone, is my all-purpose canine correction. It means to my dogs, "Stop whatever you are doing!" It is "dog talk," and all canines immediately understand it.

Follow-through makes a difference, too. If a wolf pup ignores an adult's warning growl, the adult escalates the correction into an angry snarl, a bite, or even a fight. I'm not suggesting that you have a growling and biting tussle with your dog! But observations of this behavior have taught me that a canine correction is only effective if it is enforced. Otherwise you are teaching your dog that he is free to ignore you—and that you are not really in charge.

Praise Is Important, Too

Consistency and good timing are as important with praise as they are with corrections. Too often, owners are quick to correct but not quick to reward desirable behaviors. When your dog is doing something right, let him know! For example, when he picks up his own toy and chews on it, praise him. When he eliminates outdoors, praise him. With consistent praise, these good behaviors will soon turn into reliable habits.

Here is an example. If your dog ignores your growl to stop chewing the rug, do you give up and walk away? Pack leaders do not! You can walk closer to the dog and growl again. You can grasp the scruff of the dog's neck and growl. You can physically remove the dog from the corner of the rug. Or you can roll up the rug and store it away. Some or all of these steps may be needed to solve the problem. But as pack leader you must enforce your rule: no rug chewing. By doing so you are not only preventing an unwanted behavior, you are communicating to your dog in a canine way that you are in charge.

Think about your own level of consistency. Try to improve it if you are having problems with respect and obedience from your dog. This is especially important if your dog has a dominant personality. But remember, there is no need to beat the dog into submission. Nothing about proper corrections (and follow-through) is violent or harsh.

Good timing

The timing of these corrections is significant. Think about the example above of mother dog growling at her pups even *before* they pounced on her or nipped her legs. She knew what they were about to do, but her growl told them, "Don't even think about it!" Her exquisite timing had a double effect. One, it showed that she was paying attention to the pups and that their behavior was constantly being monitored (a good pack-leader trait).

Two, it stopped a problem behavior before it even happened. Her growl did *not* mean "Stop that painful chewing." She did not let them chew on her for a while and then tell them to stop. The pups never even got the chance to misbehave! Imagine how much quicker they learned to completely avoid chewing on mom. Her good timing made the difference.

Good timing with corrections is an important pack-leader trait, but it is also a key element in obedience training. How quickly your dog learns to avoid unwanted behaviors will depend a great deal on it. A correction that comes even ten seconds after an unwanted behavior is too late! The dog may cower or "look sorry" while you yell and carry on about the chewed rug, which you found some time after the deed was done. But he will not associate his misdeed with your corrections. If you want to teach him to avoid chewing the rug, supervise him closely and correct him ("Nhaa!") when he is doing it. Better yet, correct him when he is walking toward the rug and looking at that interesting frayed corner. Your well-timed "Nhaa!" will be understood perfectly well: "Don't even think about it."

Body language

Dogs are generally attuned to the position and stance of those around them. You can use the importance of body language to help establish your pack leadership with your new dog. Some details of body language are described in the previous chapter. A few other tips are included here.

Lying down is a submissive body position for a dog. In fact, rolling over "belly up" is about the most submissive thing a canine can do. In the wild, it signals to a wolf that a combatant in a fight gives up. It usually prevents the winner from continuing the attack and even killing the loser.

For this reason, the obedience exercise Down-Stay (see Chapter 23) is a wonderful, subtle way to communicate your pack leader role. It helps keep your dog under control in all sorts of settings while at the same time reinforcing the fact that you are in charge. When I really need to get a reminder across to my dogs about who's the pack leader, I stand next to them during a Down-Stay.

Status has its privileges. The best spot on the sofa, a place on the bed, and the front seat of the car are the domain of the pack leader. Should your dog share them with you? It depends if the dog is challenging you in any way. If he growls when told to move over on the couch, you have a pack-leadership problem. In my house, that dog would no longer have couch privileges. He would need, in addition to training, many subtle reminders that I am in charge.

Here are some examples. The dog should be made to go through doorways *after* the pack leader. The Sit-Stay obedience exercise will help with this. The dog should eat *after* the family has dined. A challenging dog should wait for permission to jump in and out of the car.

These subtleties, which are all associated in some way with body status, will help you establish your pack leadership role.

Taking Charge

Your adopted dog must learn at least a moderate level of good behavior if he is going to stay in your home. Destroying your furniture, eliminating on your rugs, grabbing your kids' toys, and jumping on your guests are not the kinds of things that make for a well-loved pet. If you don't have it in you to take a pack-leadership role and to fairly and humanely correct your dog's problems, you will end up living with a nightmare. Or your adopted dog will end up back at the pound, homeless again. So do both of you a favor—take charge!

Chapter 8

Bonding from Day One

I MAKE FRIENDS WITH DOGS easily. It does not matter if the dog is an eight-week-old puppy, an adopted adolescent, an adult, or a canine senior citizen. Dogs and I like each other. This is because I am able to look at life the way they do—from a canine point of view. When I want to bond with a dog, I am willing to spend time with a dog doing what dogs like to do.

Here are some examples. Dogs like to hunt, so I take them hunting. They like to eat, so I share food with them. Dogs are extremely social animals, so I allow them to meet new people and other dogs. Dogs also need security and structure. I help them to feel secure in my home, and I develop a predictable daily routine.

Like all canines, adopted dogs need a pack leader that they can trust and take direction from. They also need to be a useful member of a pack. And all dogs need a job to do. I become pack leader and make my dogs feel vital to the pack by giving them a sense of purpose. I do this by obedience-training them.

Bonding experiences with your newly adopted dog can take many forms. And bonding also may take time, depending on your dog's age, personality, and history. But there is a lot you can do to help. This chapter will suggest things you can do to bond with your newest friend. Do as many as you can as often as you can—in no particular order. Before long, your newest friend will become your best friend!

Hunting, or the Next Best Thing

You do not have to literally go out and kill or capture other animals in order to satisfy your dog's hunting drive. Long hikes on the beach or in the woods simulate a canine hunt. *You* may be strolling, but your dog is hunting. Dogs love this. Sniffing out scent and just generally "mooking around" with the pack leader will make almost any dog very happy.

If your adopted dog is not ready for off-leash journeys (see Chapter 24, "Come on Command"), or if you live in a city environment with no access to hiking adventures, do not despair. Leash walks will work fine, but two laps around your block night after night are boring. Put your dog on the leash and explore someplace new. The togetherness of an adventure—even a mini one—is the key to a bonding experience.

Food Sharing

In my experience, it is truly a toss-up whether a dog would rather eat or hunt. If you put the two together, you will be on the fast track to creating a new canine buddy.

I always carry a supply of doggie biscuits in my pocket or backpack on a dog hike. During the hike, I sporadically call my dog to me and give him a piece of biscuit. Doing this will help your dog form a positive association with you. It will also reinforce an important obedience skill: coming when called.

Once or twice during a hike I pick a comfortable spot to take a rest. I call my dog and have him lie down next to me. I give him a biscuit or two while I pet and talk to him. My goal is for these little adventures to be something that my dog loves and looks forward to.

Car Rides

Most dogs love to go. They really do not care where, just as long as they get to go. If it is convenient and safe, take your dog with you in the car when you run errands. If you stop for a quick snack, it is okay to share a piece of your cheeseburger with your dog—another example of food in the bonding process.

Whenever you decide to bring your dog in the car, make sure that the weather is neither too hot nor too cold for his safety. Hot weather is extremely dangerous to a dog in a car. Even in shady spots with the windows partially open, a car can quickly heat up and become unsafe. Dogs have a higher body temperature than humans, and they can only perspire through their tongues and the pads of their feet. For these reasons a dog can heat up quickly and will not cool down as easily as a human. *Never* leave your dog in a car on a warm day, even for a short period of time.

Most dogs can handle cold weather if they are sheltered from the wind. Nevertheless you must use common sense when leaving your dog in a car on extremely cold days. Certainly some breeds can deal with the cold better than others can. A Siberian husky may not mind an hour in a cold car. A greyhound left under the same conditions could die.

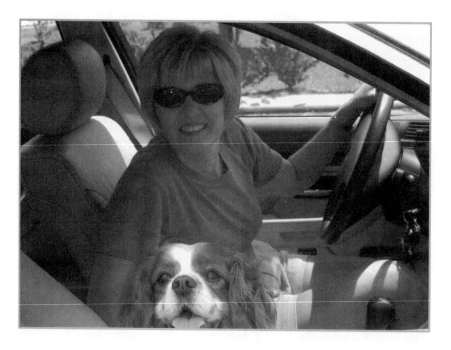

Off to another adventure together! Bonding with your adopted dog can take many forms, but there is one common element: spending time together.

A good rule of thumb to avoid tragedy and to keep car rides a fun experience is to never leave your dog in the car when weather is extreme. As you grab your car keys, do not let your dog's cute face and sad-eyed expression convince you to go against your better judgment. Your dog doesn't know when it's safe to come along, but you do. When in doubt, keep your dog safe by leaving him at home.

Also, be aware that dogs are sometimes stolen out of cars. Mall parking lots or any public place where you cannot keep an eye on your vehicle for extended periods of time should be avoided.

Socialization

If you feel confident that your adopted dog is friendly with other dogs, help him to make some canine pals. Get a dog-owning friend or two to join you on a dog hike in the woods or a leash walk through the city. This is something that your dog will learn to look forward to if you do it regularly.

You will see that your dog will come to think of these other dogs and people as part of his extended pack. An extended pack is made up of individuals that do not share the same den but come together to hunt and socialize. Their presence will help your dog's sense of belonging to a canine community of sorts, and it will help reinforce his bond to you.

Dog parks

Many cities and suburbs have dog parks. Dog parks are designated areas where people can exercise and socialize their dogs. These parks are a great way for dogs and dog people to connect. Friendships are made, training and dog care ideas are exchanged, and every once in a while two packs decide to merge. Hey, you never know what will happen at a dog park!

Get to know your adopted dog awhile before you venture to a dog park with lots of dogs. Is your adoptee dog-aggressive? (That is, does your dog pick fights with other dogs?) A crowded field of playful, running dogs may stimulate aggressive behavior in some individuals.

Neutering and obedience training may help. On the other hand, an overly submissive or easily frightened dog or an old dog may be overwhelmed by all the noise and activity. Common sense should tell you if a dog park is a good choice for your dog's outdoor play.

Be sure your dog is fully protected against diseases (by vaccinations), parasites (by flea and tick products), and unwanted sexual encounters (by spaying and neutering) before you frequent dog parks. Interaction with lots of dogs can be fun, but it is also a good avenue for trouble. If you can't seem to avoid the canine bully or the insistent Romeo or the flea-infested street waif, pick another park. These outings should be fun, not stressful, for you and your dog.

Setting Household Rules

Doing things with your new dog outside of the house is a great way to help create a bond. But just as important is making your adopted dog feel happy and secure at home. The best ways to do this are to provide your dog with leadership by setting household rules and to give him a predictable daily routine.

Making your dog behave and adhere to household rules is not going to stop him from liking you. In fact, just the opposite is true. If you make your dog behave properly by being firm, loving, and consistent, he is going to think of you as pack leader.

Decide early on what the rules of the house will be. Be sure your spouse, roommates, and children know what these rules are. Consistency from all household members will help your dog learn them quickly. For example, if everyone knows that the dog may not get on the living-room furniture or run loose in the neighborhood or eat dinner before 4 p.m., then there's a good chance those things won't happen too often.

But enforcement is an important part of this. There are few better ways to show a dog that you are *not* in charge than by being inconsistent. If one day you yell at the dog for sleeping on the good couch but the next day let him spend the morning curled up there, you are hurting your dog in two ways. One, you are confusing him. How can he behave properly when he is not clear what behaviors are okay? Two, you are letting your inconsistency show him that you are not really in charge. Dogs love and respect their pack leader more than any other individual. Be a good one by setting household guidelines and then enforcing them.

Handle your pack-leader role with care, however. People who are harsh, tyrannical, and inconsistent make dogs distrust them. If your dog does not trust you, it will be impossible to build a loving bond. Firmness and fairness are reasonable to a dog. A master–slave relationship is not.

Sharing the den

A closely knit canine pack sleeps curled up together. Doing so helps pack members to feel connected to each other. It is not necessary that you allow you newly adopted dog to sleep in bed with you—even if he did so in his previous home. (This is your house with your rules.) However, I do recommend that he sleep in your bedroom.

If your dog has destructive chewing problems or is not housebroken, I suggest that you set up an appropriate-size kennel crate in your bedroom. Otherwise, a dog nest near your bed will do. From a canine point of view, denning together at night will go a long way toward helping your dog feel that he is a part of your pack.

Obedience Training

Obedience training is essential to developing a satisfying human-canine bond. There are all sorts of positive benefits. The most obvious benefit is having a well-behaved dog that you can control and enjoy wherever you go. Dog ownership is a joy when you have a great dog.

Another benefit of obedience training is that it provides dogs with the opportunity to use their brain in a constructive way. This is necessary in order to prevent dogs from becoming bored. Boredom is one of the leading causes of behavioral problems in dogs. Bored dogs tend to chew destructively, dig holes in the yard, and bark nonstop. These are just a few of the many undesirable behaviors that drive owners to place dogs in shelters. It is possible that not having a constructive way to channel mental energy is what caused your adopted dog to be given away in the first place.

And obedience training enhances bonding, which is so important with adopted dogs. All of that practice, all of that time spent together, all of that leadership you provide—these are threads that weave together and form a dog's devotion, bonding, and even love for a new owner.

Part Three

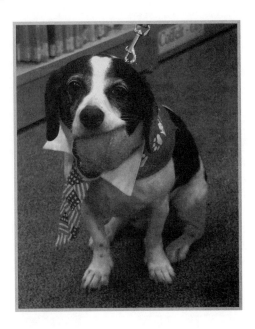

Problem Solving for Your Adopted Dog

Adopted dogs often have "issues." These may be failed housebreaking, destructive chewing, obsessive barking, separation anxiety, or fear biting. Some adopted dogs are scarred by neglect or abuse. Don't give up on your adopted dog because of such problems. They can be solved or managed successfully with the help of these chapters.

Chapter 9

Housebreaking an Adolescent or Adult Dog

MANY DOGS END UP in shelters and pounds because they were not properly housebroken. It is easy to understand why most people find it impossible to live with a dog that is urinating and defecating all over their house.

Because of this common scenario, many adopted dogs bring a housebreaking problem into their new homes. At best, adoptive owners will know that housebreaking is needed with their new dog and will be prepared from day one to deal with it. Shelter workers, breed rescue volunteers, veterinarians, or anyone who has contact with the dog may be able to identify a housebreaking problem. Sometimes previous owners point out housebreaking difficulties when the dog is given up. On the other hand, you may discover your adopted dog's secret the hard way, with a puddle on your favorite rug or an unpleasant "gift" behind the sofa.

Why is housebreaking so hard?

Most puppy owners are successful with housebreaking their young dogs, with minimal effort and few accidents. Are they just lucky? Not usually. Housebreaking success almost always depends on using a reliable training system and constant puppy supervision. The key word here is "puppy." Most young dogs with no previous bathroom habits can quickly learn housebreaking skills. It is the adopted dogs that are no longer puppies that typically have problems. Often these dogs were not properly housebroken in the first place, and they have to "unlearn" some bad habits in addition to learning good ones.

In a small number of cases, individual dogs are extremely difficult to housebreak, despite good training and supervision. In my experience, this is somewhat breed-related. For example, my records of clients and their dogs show that bichons frises are often difficult to housebreak, even as puppies. Many dachshunds require really persevering owners to achieve reliable housebreaking. This is not to say that every bichon or dachsie will make housebreaking a major task. However, my statistics show that they tend to be more of challenge. If you have adopted one of these breeds, be prepared for the possibility that housebreaking will take extra effort. The guidelines in this chapter will greatly improve your odds of success.

Early life experiences

Early environmental experiences, happening before the age of eight weeks, may influence a dog's housebreaking. Unfortunately, it is hard to know what those experiences were, especially with an adopted dog. But it is worth understanding some of these early influences, because it points out where problems may have begun.

For example, puppies born in a warm climate or during summer months may be given the opportunity to urinate and defecate outdoors at an early age. When this happens, owners have a head start on housebreaking. On the other hand, when young puppies "do their business" indoors on carpeted areas, future housebreaking is often more difficult. This happens because some breeders (or anyone caring for a puppy litter) are either unconcerned about the mess or are unaware of a puppy's early learning capabilities.

Breeders are not the only culprits. Puppies that come from pet stores are often quite difficult to housebreak. When puppies spend weeks urinating and defecating in their sleeping areas, the instinct to keep a den space clean becomes weakened. When this instinct is intact, puppies will move away from their sleeping and living area to relieve themselves. But in a pet store a puppy's full-time living space is a cage. The cage is designed so that the puppy's urine and feces fall into a compartment below. However, this is irrelevant to the puppy, because he is still eliminating in his living space. The odor permeates the puppy and conditions him to ignore the smell. Under these conditions some puppies are literally trained to be dirty.

You may or may not be able to find out if your adopted dog spent any time in a pet-store environment. Eliminating in a kennel crate may be a clue that he did. Your job of housebreaking may take a little longer. More important, you will have to be extra-diligent in following the housebreaking system outlined in this chapter.

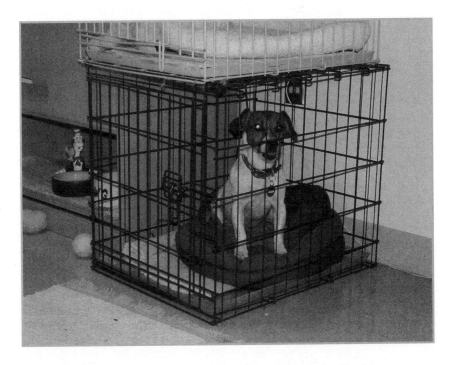

Dogs typically do not soil the place where they sleep. This is what makes a kennel crate such an ideal tool for teaching housebreaking, even to an adolescent or adult.

Owners are the main reason that dogs fail

While breed-specific difficulties and early environmental influences can contribute to housebreaking difficulties, the vast majority of young dogs that are not housebroken are victims of bad training. Too many owners rely on outdated training methods, such as starting with indoor paper training or rubbing a dog's nose in his excrement. These "techniques" are based on old wives' tales and are ineffective at best and often quite cruel. Owners who do not have a proven housebreaking system are practically doomed to failure. Supervision and a structured den area, along with effective training methods, are essential for success, especially when curing problems in an adolescent or adult.

One memorable dog that I worked with provides a great example of housebreaking mistakes and the efforts needed to correct them. This dog's owners made a lot of classic mistakes. But the dog also responded beautifully to good training. Follow this tale, and you will know how to succeed with your dog, too.

A Case Study: Lucy, the West Highland Terrier

I met Lucy in Seal Beach, California. She was about fourteen months old when I was hired to help train her. Her owners were a family of five. Mrs. Baron was a stay-at-home mom, and her husband was a successful attorney. The children, two boys and a girl, ranged from fifteen to seven years old.

I did five private lessons with the Baron family for five consecutive weeks. Mrs. Baron wanted a late-afternoon time slot so that the children could participate after school. Unfortunately, the kids really weren't too interested in training Lucy. The teenage daughter acted as though she were being punished. She just sat and stared at the ground. The middle child fidgeted and whined that he was hungry throughout the entire lesson. The littlest boy spent most of his time grabbing at Lucy or standing on his head.

Mom spent the entire lesson nagging at the kids. "Pay attention to Mr. Ross and stop acting like idiots!" Then she would keep asking me how to stop Lucy from urinating and defecating all over her house. Whenever I tried to answer her question, she would go into a trance and start looking at her watch. It was clear that these owners were not very committed to training their dog.

This scenario repeated itself every week for five weeks. Every word I said about housebreaking went in one ear and right out the other. Lucy was never supervised. She was not taken outside and given a chance to relieve herself at the appropriate times. She was not put in her kennel crate when the family left the house. Every week I patiently outlined a housebreaking system. Every week Mrs. Baron said, "Do you understand what Mr. Ross is telling us, children? We have to watch Lucy and take her out." But I knew that the minute I pulled out of the driveway, it would be business as usual at the Baron residence.

I had mixed emotions at the end of lesson five. Part of me was relieved that my commitment was over and that I no longer had to talk to a blank wall every week. On the other hand, part of me was sad and discouraged. My expertise and advice were ignored. Lucy was not given the opportunity to reach her highest potential, and I suspected that her future with this family was not very bright.

Two weeks after our last lesson, Mrs. Baron called. The conversation went something like this:

"I just came home from shopping, and Lucy pooped and peed all over my antique rugs!"

"Why wasn't Lucy in her kennel crate while you were out?"

"Well, my daughter was supposed to be right home from school and I left her a note to take Lucy out."

"I do not know what to say. You have to be consistent. If you don't stick with the system that I outlined, Lucy will never become housebroken."

"Please, Mr. Ross, would you take her and housebreak her for us?"

I explained to Mrs. Baron that if I took Lucy to my house, she would never have an accident from day one, because I would not give her the opportunity to make a mistake. I would employ my housebreaking system and stick to it. I also told Mrs. Baron that even if I kept Lucy for three weeks and she never had one accident in my house, the minute that she got home she would go back to her old routine—if given the chance. Even after Lucy returned home, the Barons would have to stick with the housebreaking system to reinforce good habits. I advised Mrs. Baron that she might as well save time and money and do the job herself. But she begged me to please do it for her. I gave in.

A Housebreaking System for Any Dog of Any Age

The first thing I did when I brought Lucy to my house was to bring her to the area in my yard where I wanted her to eliminate. This was before we even walked in the front door. I walked Lucy around the area on her leash. As she sniffed around, I repeated, "Lucy, do your business." (You can use any phrase that feels comfortable.) After about ten minutes Lucy had not eliminated, so I brought her inside the house.

Freedom is allowed only after you see the dog eliminate outside

A common mistake that new owners make is to let their dog wander freely around, exploring the new home. I did not do this. I put Lucy right into her kennel crate, which I had set up in the TV room. I did not crate Lucy to punish her because she had not eliminated outside. I crated her because I knew that she would not urinate or defecate in her crate. This is because dogs view their crate as their den area and are motivated to keep it clean.

A new pack member?

My golden retriever, Woody, had been sleeping in my office. When I let him out he ran over and checked out the new girl houseguest in the crate. Woody liked terriers, and they seemed interested in each other. After they had sniffed each other for a bit, I took

Woody out to his designated bathroom area. He knew just what to do.

The rotation system

After I came back inside with Woody, I sat and read the paper for about fifteen minutes. Then I took Lucy outside again to her designated bathroom area and walked her on the leash, back and forth. I kept repeating, "Lucy, do your business." After about five minutes she squatted and urinated. I praised her warmly: "Good girl, Lucy! Good girl!" I brought her back into the house.

Empty bladder = supervised freedom in the house

This time I did not crate her. I knew that Lucy had just emptied her bladder and that chances were very slim that she would have an accident in the house. Nevertheless, Lucy did not have complete freedom indoors. I closed two doors that led into the hall toward the bedrooms. I also closed the door to the small bathroom off the kitchen. As a result, Lucy was confined to the TV room and the kitchen. Perfect. While I made my lunch, I was able to keep a close eye on her.

Get outside: after play, naps, eating, or drinking

Lucy spent the next forty-five minutes sniffing around, checking out her new environment, playing a little with Woody, and lapping up a few slurps of water. I made both dogs lie down and stay at my feet while I ate lunch. After the last morsel of my sandwich was gone, both Lucy and Woody nodded off for a short nap.

That afternoon I had a private dog lesson scheduled. Shortly after I finished my lunch I clipped the leash to Lucy's collar and took her outside to her bathroom area. After a few minutes of walking back and forth, Lucy urinated. "Good girl, Lucy. Good girl," I said.

———

When you cannot supervise, it's crate time

When I brought Lucy indoors, I put her into the crate and headed off to my dog lesson. Woody knew the routine, so he got on his dog nest. I was gone for about two hours.

No more than four hours in the crate

I make it a point to never crate a dog or puppy for longer than four hours without a break. Most young puppies, up until around five months old, cannot go for more than four or five hours during the daytime without having to urinate or defecate. Making a puppy hold it for longer than that is unfair and counterproductive to housebreaking.

If a puppy is confined for too long he is eventually going to eliminate in the crate. This can create the same problems that occur with the pet-store puppy. If your puppy continuously soils his den area, he will learn to accept being dirty.

Even older dogs should not ever be crated for more than four hours. They should be given at least an hour break to stretch their legs and to eliminate outdoors. If a work schedule does not allow an owner to get home to give the dog a break, it is the owner's responsibility to make some kind of arrangement with someone that can. A friend, neighbor, relative, or even a professional pet sitter can be hired to do the job. It is important that this step not be overlooked. Responsible crate use—and housebreaking success—depend on it.

Consistency is the key

When I returned home from my dog lesson, the first thing I did was to take Lucy outside to her designated bathroom area. I did not let Woody out at the same time, because I did not want him to be a distraction to Lucy. Lucy seemed to be catching on already. After just a few minutes of our bathroom ritual she urinated. Still no poops, however.

I was not too concerned about this. When I had picked Lucy up that morning, Mrs. Baron told me that she had pooped in the dining room right after breakfast. Since Lucy had not eaten dinner yet, I assumed that she did not need to move her bowels again.

The dog can be quick, but the attentive owner must be quicker

I kept Lucy on her leash in the yard while Woody came outside to relieve himself. After he was finished I brought both dogs inside and again gave Lucy supervised freedom. While I looked through my mail the two dogs poked around the TV room.

I kept glancing over at Lucy, keeping an eye on what she was doing. All of a sudden when I looked up I did not see Lucy. I quickly came around the kitchen counter to find Lucy about to squat.

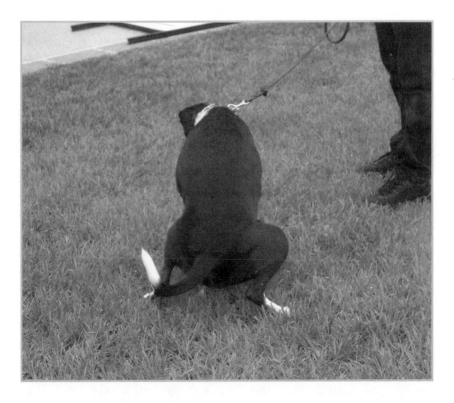

Make sure you observe your dog eliminating outdoors. Sending him outside and assuming he emptied out is not good enough for housebreaking success.

Well-timed corrections

I immediately corrected Lucy with a firm, guttural "Nhaa!" She froze. I calmly walked over to her, picked her up, found her leash, and headed outside. Once outdoors I clipped the leash to Lucy's collar, put her down, and quickly walked her to the bathroom area.

After about two minutes of repeating "Lucy, do your business," she pooped. Yay! "Good girl, Lucy! Good girl!" I said enthusiastically. (Isn't it amazing what we dog owners can get excited about?) Lucy and I walked around for a few more minutes, and she squatted and urinated. "Good girl, Lucy!" I picked her up and kissed her cute white face all the way to the house. Once inside, Lucy was again allowed supervised freedom. I knew she had emptied out, so there was minimal chance of a mistake.

To correct or not to correct

In the scene described above, I spotted Lucy as she was *about* to make a mistake. I corrected her with a guttural growl. It is okay and even worthwhile to correct a dog for urinating or defecating in the house. However, the timing must be perfect, and the correction must be appropriate.

Remind yourself that the only time it is ever justifiable to correct a housebreaking accident is if you catch the dog about to eliminate or in the process of eliminating. Ten seconds after the fact is too late. Your dog may cower or act fearful if you scold and carry on after finding a puddle on the floor. But your dog will not associate your corrections with the *act of making the mistake*. Consider what the Barons did when Lucy messed up.

Late corrections do no good and a lot of harm

Mrs. Baron told me that she never caught Lucy urinating or defecating in the house. She always found the mess after the fact. Unfortunately, she either did not hear or did not believe my advice about proper timing of corrections. She would drag Lucy to the mess (sometimes hours after the deed was done), show it to her, and yell, "Bad girl! Look what you did! Bad girl!"

These poorly timed corrections did achieve a few things. They taught Lucy to distrust her owner, because from Lucy's point of view all the yelling and scolding seemed completely random and unpredictable. They also taught Lucy to become apprehensive at the sight of a pile of poop or a puddle of urine.

Mrs. Baron incorrectly interpreted Lucy's apprehensive behavior as guilty behavior. This led Mrs. Baron to conclude that Lucy knew she had done something wrong. In fact, Mrs. Baron believed that Lucy was eliminating in the house because she was a bad, spiteful dog. Nothing could have been further from the truth.

Proper timing with corrections would have improved Lucy's behavior considerably. Lucy would have understood exactly when she was making a mistake. And with consistent handling she would soon have learned not to make those mistakes again. But proper timing is impossible without supervision. If you are not watching your dog you cannot affect her behavior.

Develop a pattern and stick with it

As our first day together was winding down, I continued my housebreaking system with Lucy into the evening. If she urinated when I took her out, I gave her supervised freedom in the house. If she did not urinate, I crated her when we went back inside.

At 6 p.m. I fed her dinner. Sometime within the next hour I expected her to defecate. So every fifteen minutes I took her outside to her area. I kept rotating her from the crate to her outside bathroom area until she finally pooped. At seven I left the house for an evening dog lesson. Two hours later when I returned I took Lucy outside. She both urinated and defecated! Eureka!

Eight bedtime hours in the crate is okay

That night I went to bed at eleven o'clock. Before turning in, I took Lucy out and she urinated. I brought her in and moved her kennel crate into my bedroom. My plan was to keep Lucy in her crate all night long. If she woke up in the middle of the night and cried, I would take her outside to her bathroom area. However, I did not anticipate that happening. During sleeping hours a dog's metabolism slows down, and the dog will need to urinate and defecate less often.

Sure enough, Lucy slept though the night. So did Woody and I. We were all extremely exhausted. Housebreaking a dog is a lot of work!

First thing the next morning I immediately took Lucy to her outside bathroom area. She did a rather large morning pee and came in for breakfast. After breakfast, back outside. It took three or four rotations from the crate to the yard before Lucy defecated. When she did, she was praised warmly and earned supervised freedom in the house.

Our day two went pretty much like day one with the exception of the housebreaking correction. Lucy did not attempt to pee or poop in the house. When I left the house I crated her. When I was home I took her out every hour. She was already starting to get the hang of quickly urinating when I took her to the outdoor spot.

A big breakthrough, but I did not rest

On Lucy's eighth day with me, at about six o'clock in the evening, I was sitting on the sofa watching a baseball game. The dogs had just finished their dinner. I was watching an exciting play at second base and was planning to take Lucy outside to the bathroom area.

I looked up and there was Lucy standing by the back door "telling" me that she needed to go out. "Good girl, Lucy!" (I'll catch the game highlights later.) I clipped the leash to Lucy's collar and hustled her right to her area. She immediately urinated. "Good girl, Lucy. Good girl." She sniffed around a minute more and then pooped. "Good girl, Lucy. You are such a good girl." Lucy was getting it. I was so proud of her! But one good moment does not mean that the job is done.

Consistency will pay off

It took eight days of our bathroom routine for Lucy to indicate to me that she wanted to get outside when she needed to relieve herself. This was great, because it indicated that a behavior pattern had been established. But this did *not* mean that the behavior pattern was an infallible habit. Keep in mind that Lucy had been urinating and defecating primarily indoors for a year. A yearlong habit is not going to be extinguished in eight days. It was not going to be extinguished in three or four weeks even. For an old behavior to be eradicated, I believe that a new behavior has to be consistently repeated for as long as the old behavior existed. This means that Lucy's owners had to be prepared for many months of sticking with this housebreaking system.

Adopted dogs have an advantage

The one advantage that Lucy did have going for her was her age. Young puppies do not have much control over their bowels or bladders until they are at least four months old. This means that an owner with a young puppy will need to take the puppy outside more often throughout the day and even during the night. And yes, it is exhausting and inconvenient. But the alternative is worse, as the Barons discovered. A chronic house-soiler is not the kind of pet anyone wants to live with.

If your adopted dog is an adolescent or adult, he will have the advantage of more bodily control. This will allow you to go back and forth to the yard fewer times each day and probably not at all during the night. Also, your home is full of new sights, sounds, smells, and routines to your dog. Use your dog's adjustment period to your home as an opportunity to establish new behaviors right from the start. It will be one more way that you can increase your odds for success.

Time flies when you are having fun

My three weeks with Lucy were over before I knew it. As I had predicted to Mrs. Baron, Lucy did not have any housebreaking accidents in my home during her stay. This is not to say that she was housebroken. I had only established a behavior pattern. If this behavior pattern was going to be turned into a lifetime habit, it would have to be repeated consistently for a much longer period. Because Lucy had been urinating and defecating in the house for a year, it could take that long to form a new habit.

A controlled environment

In the Barons' defense, I did have several advantages. Besides having the experience of training other dogs with this housebreaking system, I lived in a much smaller house than the Baron family. This made it easier to supervise Lucy closely. I could close doors and put up baby gates, limiting Lucy's access only to rooms where I would be.

Also, because I lived alone I did not have to contend with other people interfering with my training routine. It is essential that everyone in a multiperson household be at least aware of an ongoing housebreaking program. Ideally, teens and other adults can help so that one handler does not give up from exhaustion. Just be sure that all helpers are prepared to do it right.

No matter what success I had, the Baron family still would need to pick up where I left off by sticking with the training schedule that I had established. If they did not, Lucy's doggie housebreaking vacation at my house would be a waste of everyone's time and money.

The Barons' Year-Long Task

When I brought Lucy home, she was excited to see her house. However, before I even let her into the Barons' house to reunite with her family, I took her to her designated bathroom area in the backyard. It took several minutes of my repeating Lucy's bathroom mantra before she squatted and urinated. When she did I praised her warmly.

Lucy was very happy to see her family. They, too, were excited to see Lucy. Even the teenage daughter greeted her enthusiastically. Lucy raced around the kitchen and family room with a case of "puppy crazies." Each family member gave her hugs and pats. After fifteen minutes of exuberant greetings and conversation, I decided that Lucy had better make another trip outside.

Mrs. Baron accompanied me. I had her walk Lucy around the bathroom area, repeating, "Lucy, do your business." Lucy kept looking over at me. Finally I chimed in, "Lucy, do your business," and she squatted and urinated. Lucy was used to my voice.

However, if the Barons stuck with it, Lucy would adjust to their verbal tones.

It's my job, so I'll say it again

When we came back inside I sat the Baron family down for a talk. I explained that there was only one way that Lucy would form a habit of using a specific outdoor area at the Barons' home. That was if the Barons would take over where I left off. *They had to stick with the system.* If they fell back into their old inconsistent ways, Lucy would go back to her old ways, too.

I told them that in Lucy's case it could take up to a year of consistency to extinguish the old behavior of soiling in the house and to establish a new habit of urinating and defecating outside. They all agreed to try. I crossed my fingers for luck.

If only life were a Lassie episode

Unfortunately, things do not always turn out exactly the way we would like them to. A couple of months after I had returned Lucy, I received a short letter in the mail from the Barons. Life with Lucy had not worked out. The very next afternoon after she returned home, Lucy had defecated on the living-room rug. The teenage daughter had received a phone call and forgot to keep an eye on the dog.

The Barons' veterinarian had found a home for Lucy with an older couple. Apparently things were going well, and the couple loved Lucy. Mrs. Baron gave them the written training information that I had provided, and they were having no problem teaching Lucy to eliminate outside. Mrs. Baron thanked me in her letter for my help and said that when they got another puppy, they would call me. She also said that the next time they would try a different breed that was easier to train.

After reading their note, all I could do was let out a large sigh. Lucy's breed wasn't the problem. Neither was her age. Lucy's housebreaking problems were caused by her owners' failure to stick with an effective training system. Lucy's unmistakable success in my home and with her second owners did not surprise me at all. She was a healthy, sweet, bright little dog. When she was shown what to do and was prevented from making mistakes, Lucy soon developed a pattern of doing the right thing. I have seen a great many adolescent and adult dogs achieve housebreaking success. If you stick with this training system, you have every reason to feel optimistic that your adopted dog will succeed, too.

Troubleshooting

A lot of what can go wrong with housebreaking is captured here in my tale of Lucy and her family. A few other problems deserve some mention.

Ill health may present a difficult obstacle to housebreaking success. Some ailments, such as a urinary-tract infection, may cause your dog to urinate every ten or twenty minutes. An intestinal blockage can prevent bowel movements altogether. These conditions are not normal and should not be viewed as a housebreaking challenge. They are veterinary problems that need prompt attention. As with people, a noticeable change in bathroom habits can indicate illness. Do not delay in seeking veterinary help.

An elderly dog may lose bladder and/or bowel control. If medical intervention cannot help, adjust the dog's environment so that soiling is contained to an area that can be easily and frequently cleaned up. Spread newspapers or washable rugs in the dog room or around your dog's bed. Until you decide euthanasia is needed (or the dog dies a natural death), keep him as clean and comfortable as you possibly can.

"Submissive urination" is a term that describes the problem of "peeing whenever he's excited." It is not a housebreaking problem, because the dog cannot control it. In fact, many dogs that urinate submissively do not even realize that they are releasing urine. Ways to handle this annoying but not disastrous problem are discussed in Chapter 14, "Shy and Submissive Dogs."

Both males and females may urinate indoors as a way to mark territory. This is a frustrating problem, because these dogs may otherwise seem to have good housebreaking skills. For some reason the scent of a certain railing post, sofa corner, or doorway inspires these dogs to pee. You can try a few things, the first of which is spaying or neutering. Any dog with a healthy dose of reproductive hormones flowing in his or her veins will be prone to this behavior. Read Chapter 31, "Spaying and Neutering Myths," if you need more convincing of the many benefits of this surgery.

I would handle a dog that marked indoors mostly as an unhousebroken individual. Strict crating might not be needed, but careful supervision is. Keep the dog in the room with you. Clean previously marked spots with an enzyme cleaner or other product designed for pet urine. Be prepared with a firm "Nhaa!" correction if you see the dog even *sniffing* around a favored spot.

Many years ago, one of my clients' dogs had the bad habit of occasionally peeing in the center of the owner's bed when he was not home. This dog was neutered and perfectly housebroken, so his behavior was puzzling and annoying. Since it only happened when the owner was not home, the dog could not be corrected with proper timing. However, the owner could change the environment to prevent the dog from getting to the bed. My recommendation was simply to close the bedroom door when the owner went out. The bottom line is that a problem like this will continue unless you take steps to stop the dog from repeating the behavior.

Postscript

My experience with the Barons was one more confirmation in my belief that pet owners must be taught to train their own dogs. Rarely have I found it effective when owners have their dogs trained for them. This is especially true with housebreaking. For the dog's entire lifetime, the owners are the ones who will be letting the dog in and out, watching for potential accidents, and monitoring what happens outdoors. If they cannot stay attuned to their own dog, I cannot do it for them.

Lucy was the last dog that I ever took into my home to help housebreak for a client. But the Barons were certainly not the last owners I taught how to do it. For every "Lucy" in my files, I have hundreds of dogs of all breeds and ages that achieved housebreaking success with their owners. By following this program, you and your adopted dog can be successful, too.

Chapter 10

Mouthing and Biting Problems

NOBODY WANTS TO LIVE with a dog that bites. If your adopted dog is a biter or even a dog that "mouths" a lot, this chapter is required reading. Your own safety plus that of your family, neighbors, and friends depends on prompt and appropriate handling of this potentially serious problem.

Mouthing is normal puppy behavior

Chewing on our hands and feet, grabbing at shirtsleeves or pant legs, nipping at our nose or ears. These are examples of mouthing. Mouthing is a form of biting that is normal behavior with almost all puppies. It is in fact a learning tool necessary to a puppy's social development.

Nevertheless, it is a behavior that most puppy owners find annoying. Fortunately, with proper training, mouthing disappears, with most puppies, at around five months of age. Although mouthing can be exasperating to deal with, it becomes a serious problem only if left unchecked. This information about mouthing will help you understand why a dog mouths and why it is so important to teach the dog to stop, no matter what its age.

"But he's only playing"

Many owners are confused about why puppies mouth. "He's just teething," they explain. Or they claim, "She's not being mean, she's just playing."

Mouthing on fellow pack members has nothing to do with teething. Puppies do not begin to loose their milk teeth until they are four months old. However, they begin mouthing and biting at around three weeks old. And left unchecked, mouthing can continue long after the puppy teeth are gone and the adult teeth are in place.

Owners are correct when they say that a puppy is not being mean when it mouths on them. Mouthing is not an indicator of bad temperament or a mean streak in a dog. But it is definitely not just playing.

Pack hierarchy

In their first weeks and months of life, young puppies bite their littermates in order to find a position in the pecking order of the pack. Wrestling, biting, growling, and competing for the best nursing position are all normal and important parts of a puppy's development. If you ever get a chance to watch a litter of puppies, do so. Unless they are sleeping or nursing, they are probably wrestling and biting on each other. These behaviors teach puppies how and when to be tough and assertive. It also teaches them when to back off and submit. Without this essential learning experience, a dog would be socially stunted.

A breeder's job

The majority of dog breeders separate littermates sometime between eight and twelve weeks of age. This is when most puppies are given away or sold to new owners. After eight to twelve weeks of observing this litter, an astute breeder has a pretty good idea of the pack ranking of each puppy. Some puppies are dominant and some are submissive. Others are somewhere in between.

Being aware of this information helps the breeder place an appropriate puppy personality type with an owner. The most dominant puppy can be placed in a family without small children, or at least with owners who have the ability to control such an assertive dog. The most submissive individual can be put into a nonintimidating setting, one that will work best with the puppy's gentler temperament.

Mother knows best

Dog breeders with a good understanding of canine behavior make it a point to leave their puppy litters in daily contact with the mother dog, right up until adoption time. This is because mother dogs play an important role in the social development of their puppies. One important way they do this is by disciplining their puppies.

As puppies grow older, mother dog stops them when they nurse too vigorously. She will growl or snap at them as if to say, "Slow down." She may get up and leave, shaking her pups loose from her teats, grumbling at them. When puppies bite at her ears or chew on her legs, she will growl and sometimes snap at the delinquent individuals. Mother dog lets her puppies know in no uncertain terms that she is the undisputed pack leader. When she tells them to stop an unwanted behavior, she makes sure that they comply.

Where do I stand?

A puppy that misses this social interaction with its mother is often a problem for new owners to train and to live with. This is particularly true if the puppy was the most dominant youngster in the litter. Mother dog's presence is profoundly important in socializing a dominant pup.

Imagine the biggest, toughest, most assertive male puppy in a litter with little or no interaction with his mother. From three weeks to ten weeks of age this dominant little pup bossed everyone in his universe around. For the majority of this puppy's short existence he ruled the roost; he never learned how or when to submit to anyone. By the time he is eight weeks old, he thinks he is invincible.

A dog of this description is a challenge for some puppy owners and a disaster for others. Many such puppies end up as shelter dogs because they were "too much to handle." It is not an uncommon scenario. The root of the problem often is the lack of proper socialization with littermates and/or the mother dog. Puppies that were placed with owners much too young (that is, before seven or eight weeks of age) are especially prone to this problem. They missed out on those important weeks of learning to respect a pack leader.

But why is mouthing a problem?

It is pretty obvious why a mouthing puppy is a problem in a human household. Those sharp little puppy teeth hurt! They also rip clothes and put bloody little holes in legs and hands.

After the needle-sharp milk teeth fall out, the adult teeth that replace them do not hurt as much. However, six-month-old puppies clamp down harder than ten-week-old puppies do. So you are only trading pinprick hurt for a bite that will easily bruise your skin. Even if your older puppy does not clamp down hard enough to bruise you, who wants a slobbery arm or shirtsleeve?

But the pain and slobber are only part of the problem. More significant is the unspoken message that you are giving a puppy when you allow him to mouth you. You are unambiguously saying to him in dog language, "You are the boss. I will follow direction from you, because you are more dominant in our pack than I am." This can only lead to trouble.

The adolescent

Puppies that are still mouthing by the time they reach the "teenage" developmental stage, which is at about one year old, are going to be hard to handle. This is particularly true if for most of their lives they have basically been doing whatever they felt like doing—whenever they felt like doing it. An adolescent dog that thinks of himself as the pack leader in a household, or at least a very dominant pack member, will not easily accept a human handler taking charge and starting obedience training.

Even if owners have been doing some obedience training with this dog, they will have problems succeeding. This is because obedience-training a dog while at the same time allowing him to mouth sends a mixed message. When you obedience-train, you are essentially saying to the dog, "I'm in charge; you must follow my direction." But allowing mouthing is saying the exact opposite to the dog: "You are more dominant. You are in charge." Inconsistency with mouthing will doom any dog-training attempts to failure.

How to Stop Your Dog from Mouthing

I curb mouthing with adolescent dogs the same way that I do with young puppies. I imitate mother dog. Whenever the puppy chewed on mother dog, she growled at him. I do the same thing. Using a guttural tone, I correct my dog with a firm "Nhaa!" every time he attempts to bite.

That does not always stop the dog. When puppies ignore their mother's growl, she will escalate her correction. She will growl louder or longer; she may growl deeper; she may grab the pup at the back of its neck. So do I. If I growl "Nhaa!" and the puppy ignores me, I grab a handful of loose skin at the nape of the puppy's neck and growl "Nhaa!" again a little louder, as I stare menacingly into the pup's eyes. My goal is to appear tough and serious, communicating with my voice and actions that I mean business. Note that I am not hitting, kicking, or harming the dog in any way to show my authority. I am using canine "language" to communicate. It is understood by every dog I have ever met.

Of course, this takes consistency in order to work. It is impossible to eliminate mouthing behavior with one mighty correction. Puppies and adolescents test their limits many times over—sometimes hundreds of times over! That's natural. Your job is to give the dog the same response every time he tries. Growl and act tough! Convince the puppy or adolescent that *every time* he puts his mouth on you, it will not be tolerated.

It helps if you get in the mindset that you are *indignant* at the very idea that your puppy thinks he can dominate you. If you are not truly indignant, fake it. Your pup must think that mouthing makes you, the pack leader, quite angry.

It does not matter if it takes twenty corrections or two thousand, mouthing must not be tolerated. Growl and correct your dog every time he tries it. If you sometimes correct mouthing and sometimes allow it, you will never succeed in eliminating it. Wishy-washiness will inspire a dominant dog to be even more persistent with mouthing, with the goal of eventually achieving dominance over you. If you take the attitude, starting today, that your dog's mouthing will be corrected every time, it truly will dissipate.

Success with this training may take time, especially if your adopted dog is an adolescent and has developed a habit of mouthing. You can still train him to stop this annoying behavior by using the same techniques. However, it will probably take longer and require more vigilance on your part. If the dog has been getting away with this behavior for nine months, it may take that long to stop it.

Mouthing the Kids

I hear from many owners that the dog does not mouth the adults but is a terror on the kids. It's easy to understand why. Kids are a pushover when it comes to canine dominance. They are smaller, easily intimidated, have high-pitched voices, and have little or no ability to give effective corrections.

This is where you come in. A mouthing dog needs a ton of supervision. If my one-year-old dog were mouthing my six-year-old daughter, I would be all over him with growls and corrections. Also, the two of them would not spend any unsupervised time together until I got the problem under control.

This may seem like an extreme way to respond to some seemingly playful puppy mouthing. It's not. Every time a dog mouths, that dog is one step closer to thinking that it is okay to put his teeth on human skin. With repetition and growing confidence, that dog can easily become a biter—one of the biggest reasons that people give up their dogs or have them euthanized. Prevention is a lot easier than a cure.

Adult Dogs That Bite

Many adult dogs that bite do so because they have been allowed by their owners to believe that they are the pack leader. I call this category of dog a protest biter. A protest biter probably does not have an inherently bad temperament. He just believes that he can bite anyone who challenges him. This is because he is convinced that he is in charge.

Dogs achieve their adult personalities at around two years old. It is usually around this age when mouthing turns into full-fledged biting. Although it is possible for puppies and adolescents to be protest biters, it is not as common. More typical is the adult biter that mouthed a lot throughout puppyhood. The dog probably also grumbled and growled whenever he was made to do things. Now that he is an adult, if you get in his way, he will bite you.

Once your dog reaches this stage you no longer have a mouthing problem. You now have a serious biting problem.

"How dare you tell me what to do," said the dog

The protest biter, in most cases, is not going to suddenly start attacking everyone in sight. He is probably going to be fine with people, as long as things are going his way. It is only when someone tries to make this dog do something he does not feel like doing that he will become vicious.

For example, try removing this individual from a sofa. He will snap at you! If you try to make him lie down or get brushed, he will bite you. Trim his toenails? He won't even let you near them. A professional groomer can help. So can the tips in this chapter, plus improving your pack-leader image, as described in Chapter 7.

Bad breeding

There are some unfortunate dogs that have inherited lousy personalities. These dogs are sometimes genetic misfits that could even be mentally unstable. This probably is a result of poor breeding. Parents or grandparents with bad personalities are usually going to produce offspring with bad personalities. I have seen it happen.

Every once in a while a puppy comes along with a nasty personality that is hard to explain. Three generations of the dog's ancestors may all have been sweet-natured dogs. But Fido, right from the beginning is a nightmare. Where did this come from? Maybe Great-Great-Uncle Fido on the mother's side was nasty. Genetics are a tricky thing. Good breeders not only breed selectively for hunting skills in the field or good looks in the show ring. They also screen ancestors many generations back for personality traits.

Socialization

Personality flaws can also be attributed to poor socialization. Puppies that were not properly socialized at an early age can become fearful of humans. Physical abuse or nutritional neglect can affect a dog's personality as well. Abused dogs often develop a suspicious nature.

Fear biting is prevalent with shy or easily spooked dogs. Such dogs will snap or bite if they do not have an opportunity to run away from a fearful situation. Dogs that are fearful and suspicious are very hard to change once they have acquired their adult personalities. Chapter 14, "Shy and Submissive Dogs," gives tips on helping these dogs.

Biting breeds?

Aggressive biting behavior can also be breed-related. There are many breeds of dog that were developed to be aggressive and vicious. Fighting breeds such as pit bulls bite and kill people every year—in fact, pit bulls do so far more than any other breed. Yet all pit bulls are not vicious. But they are statistically more dangerous than golden retrievers.

The same is true of dogs that have been selectively bred for protection. Rottweilers seem to generate headlines a little too often and are second on the list of dog-bite fatalities in the United States since 1979. They are followed by German shepherds.

I realize that these three breeds are not the only potentially danger-ous dogs. There are many. Take chow chows, for example. In my expe-rience, 98 percent of all chows are inherently grumpy dogs. I've never met one that did not try to bite me.

I am aware that it is not a politically correct stance in the dog train-ing community to blame specific breeds for bad behavior. However, I know for a fact that certain breeds of dogs are more prone to biting than others, and it would be untruthful to suggest otherwise.

Your Options

Over the past thirty years I have received hundreds of calls from peo-ple looking for help with adult dogs that were vicious. I counseled many of these owners, helping them to see what their options were and how to evaluate their choices.

In some cases all an owner needed to do was get his or her dog into obedience training in order to stop a biting problem. The dog in question may have been submissive by nature and simply spoiled. Once the owner took charge and established a pack-leader image, the dog's biting problem could be stopped. Other times it was not that simple.

Can biters be cured?

It may be possible to rehabilitate adult dogs that are dominant and have a serious biting problem. However, it is not easy. This is especially true if the dog is well into adulthood. For a dog with a long-term his-tory of biting, I believe that the prognosis for successfully stopping biting altogether is not good. Personally, I would be hesitant to com-pletely trust any dog that has a history of biting around my friends and family.

It is beyond the scope of this book to teach pet owners how to undo a serious biting problem. Some owners successfully manage their biters, keeping them faithfully away from whatever sets them off. Others try to rehabilitate the dog. There are dog trainers who special-ize in training dogs to bite—and not to bite. Owners do have the option of putting their faith and money into the hands of these specialized trainers. However, I have personally never referred anyone with a biting dog to a specific trainer. This is because I have not had a professional relationship with—or confidence in—any trainer that did this type of work. Therefore, I have always recommended that people check with their veterinarian for a referral or search other avenues for a specific name. I have always cautioned owners to thoroughly check out all trainers before getting involved with them, regardless of who recommended them.

How far should you go to rehabilitate a biter?

I do not believe that dogs should be physically abused in an attempt to train them. If you are looking into rehabilitation training, be sure to find out specifically what the trainer plans to do to rehabilitate your dog. You have to trust your sensibilities as to whether or not the means justifies the end. I would rather place a dog in a different environment or humanely euthanize him than have him abused in the name of "training."

Giving up a biting dog

There are times when I recommend that owners give up their aggressive dog that has a serious biting problem. I always hate doing this. Giving up a dog is a difficult thing to do, especially one that was adopted with the hope of giving it a better life. And no dog is 100 percent horrible.

When a serious biting incident happens, owners are often frantic and know that they have to do something. However, when old Cujo is sleeping sweetly in front of the fireplace, giving him away is the last thing that people want to think about.

Nevertheless, when the owners' safety or the welfare of their children are in question, there may be no other rational choice. Believe me, I love dogs. They are my essence! But people, particularly children, are more important. A dangerously aggressive dog does not belong in a family home. If your best efforts fail at making your adopted dog a good pet, Chapter 16 will help you decide what to do next.

_____

Chapter 11

Excessive Barking

EVERY DAY DOGS are given away or placed in shelters and pounds because they bark too much. "Too much" is the key phrase here. It is okay if your adopted dog barks, as long as the barking is not excessive and is not happening at an inappropriate time. It is *not* okay if it is happening because the dog is often alone ten or more hours a day. The fix for this is to spend more time with your dog, or to arrange for someone who can.

Barking is a normal form of canine vocal communication. Almost all canines bark. Although howling is more commonly associated with wild canines, such as the wolf and coyote, they, too, bark. However, wild canines bark much less than their domestic cousin, the dog.

Dogs bark for many reasons. They bark to get our attention. Some dogs bark to ask owners to let them in or out. They might bark to remind us that it is their mealtime. Dogs often bark to solicit play.

Dogs with a protective instinct bark to alert family members that someone is approaching the house or yard. They may bark to drive off other animals that invade what is perceived as their territory, or to release anxiety when they have been left alone and are feeling isolated.

Reasons for Excessive Barking

Social isolation is the most common reason that dogs bark excessively. When puppies are left alone, they sometimes whimper or bark nonstop. This vocal behavior may be a way to alert pack members to where they are. Dogs that are isolated in pens or tied out on runs in the backyard often bark nonstop. When dogs are placed in these situations, barking is one way to release frustration.

Any behavior that a dog repeats will eventually become a habit. If your adopted dog is a nonstop barker, it is probable that he was socially exiled in a previous environment. When a puppy spends several months or a year barking every time he is left alone, a conditioned response will develop that may last a lifetime if not corrected. The dog's cue is your leaving the house and the door closing or the sound of your car starting. His response is nonstop barking.

Built to bark

Abundant barking is also a breed characteristic. Although all breeds and mixes of breeds (with the exception of the basenji) do bark, some dogs are more prone to be bigmouths. For example, some of the herding breeds love to bark.

One of my all-time favorite dogs was my late Australian shepherd, Drifter. He was my friend and partner for many years, but boy, could his motor mouth drive you nuts. No matter what was going on, Drifter felt obliged to bark about it. A noise outside would often set him off. When he was in the car, just turning down a road to a favorite beach or hiking area would start him barking. While our Labradors would be retrieving bumpers off our backyard dock, Drifter would be racing back and forth on the dock, barking.

The Welsh corgi and Shetland sheepdog are two herding breeds that also love to bark. Barbara loves shelties and always talks about one day owning one. I agree that shelties are a great breed, except for the barking. I don't know if I can take living with another noisy herding dog.

Some of the smaller breeds are reputed to be "yappers." I have found this to be true with Yorkshire, West Highland, and Jack Russell terriers. Small poodles and dachshunds can also be quite vocal. If you own one of these breeds or a dog that is mixed with one, you probably know what I mean.

But an individual dog of almost any breed or mix of breeds can be a barker.

Quiet on Command

Barking is not a problem if your dog will be quiet on command. The best obedience exercise that I ever taught Drifter was this. Each day, Drifter would go into a frenzy of barking when the mail carrier drove by. He would bark like a maniac if a dog came into the yard. He would sound off if he heard a child on the road. Any stimulus whatsoever would set him off. However, I could live with his barking as long as I could say, "Drifter, quiet!" and he would stop. Without this command, life with Drifter probably would have been unbearable.

Teaching Quiet on Command

I attached a six-foot cloth training leash to Drifter's buckle collar and allowed him to drag it around inside the house. I was careful that he did not get it wrapped around furniture.

Whenever Drifter began to bark, I would pick up his leash, bring him over to me, and make him sit. I then held his collar with my left hand and gently grasped his muzzle with my right. The fingers of my right hand were under his muzzle, and my thumb was across the top. I gave him the command "Drifter, quiet!" in a firm, but not loud, tone.

I did not squeeze his muzzle. I just lightly and briefly held it closed. If you apply too much pressure, the dog will whimper and flag his head from side to side. Your goal is not to frighten or restrain him; it is to show him what "quiet" means.

Likewise, the purpose of holding his muzzle is not to correct him for barking. All that you are doing is teaching the dog to associate the command "Quiet" with stopping the barking. Whenever Drifter began barking and I wanted him to stop, I repeated this technique. As with all obedience training, consistency is the key.

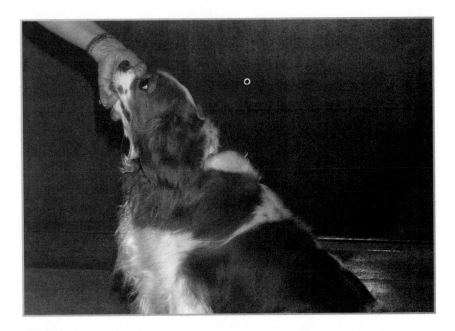

Teach your dog to be quiet on command by gently closing his mouth and saying "Quiet." Don't grip too hard or hold too long—you're not trying to squeeze the bark out!

Teach first, then test and correct

After repeating this procedure consistently for two months, I felt that Drifter had made an association between the command and response. I decided that it was reasonable to test Drifter. And if it was necessary, I was prepared to correct him.

As a correction tool I used a plastic spray water bottle, like the type used to spray houseplants. I adjusted the nozzle to a steady stream and filled it with clear, cool water. Most dogs hate a squirt in the face. It will usually startle them a bit and stop them, for a few moments, from what they are doing.

A word of caution: Do *not* use lime juice, lemon juice, white vinegar, or any other substance for this purpose. Fill your spray bottle with just plain water. Anything other than water can be irritating to your dog's eyes and should never be used.

Another word of caution: Simply spraying your dog in the face and saying "Quiet!" is usually ineffective. For this Quiet on Command training to work, it is necessary for the dog to first form an association between your command and his response. Take the time to show your dog what to do before you test and correct him.

The test

The next time Drifter started barking, I tested his understanding of our training by giving the command "Drifter, quiet!" He did stop barking for a split second. Then he thought about it and went right back to sounding off.

The correction

I gave him an abrupt squirt right on the muzzle with the plant sprayer and repeated the Quiet command. He sat, looked at me with an offended and indignant look, and let out a big sigh. He went into the other room and flopped down. I praised him: "Good boy." He didn't have to like my command; he just had to comply. And my praise rewarded him for doing so.

Consistency and practice

This scenario was repeated several times over the next couple of weeks. After a half-dozen squirts, all I had to do was show Drifter the bottle and say "Drifter, quiet!" He would stop barking and then go lie down. After a month or so I no longer needed the squirt bottle to get Drifter to obey the command. However, I did keep it around for future reinforcement, which was necessary now and then over the years.

Drifter loved to bark and heard the command "Quiet" many times throughout his fourteen years. His understanding and reliable response to the command made life with him a joy.

Nothing is perfect

One downside to the Quiet on Command exercise is that the dog does not interpret the command as "Stop barking, and I don't want to hear from you again all day." If you have a chronic barker, that may be what you were hoping for! This exercise simply teaches dogs to stop barking on command.

This means that the next time there is a sound or a sight that stimulates the dog, he is going to bark again. This can be a problem if you live in a situation where your dog is continually stimulated.

Also, Quiet on Command is effective only if you are there to give the command. What if you are not around, but your dog still barks and disturbs others? You may risk all sorts of trouble, from angry family members to eviction from your apartment.

Home Alone

If your dog is a chronic barker in your absence (or you find it a nuisance to give the command a hundred times a day), you may need to try another approach to solving your problem. Bark training collars may be the answer.

Bark training collars: how they work

A bark collar uses negative reinforcement to condition a dog to avoid barking. Simply put, the collar gives the dog a correction whenever he barks. The collar senses the sound and responds with an immediate correction.

There are three different types of corrections to choose from with bark collars. Your own sensibilities, your dog's sensitivities, and your budget will influence which one (if any) seems right for you.

That stinks!

Some bark training collars release a citronella spray when the dog barks. Most dogs intensely dislike the smell of citronella. After only a few experiences with the citronella bark collar, they learn that the unpleasant odor shows up when they bark. They learn to avoid barking. (It amazes me that dogs dislike the lemony smell of citronella but are attracted to cat poop. Go figure.)

To be sure of the safety of citronella with dogs, I checked with my favorite veterinary source. Dr. Chuck Noonan, the Animal Doctor of Weston, Connecticut, assures me that citronella spray, as used in these collars, is not harmful to dogs. The lives of my dogs have been in this vet's capable hands for many years, and I do trust his judgment.

I hate that sound!

Some bark collars correct the dog by emitting a high-pitched sound that dogs find unpleasant. The training theory is the same, only the correction is different. The dog barks and has a disagreeable experience. With repetition the dog learns to avoid barking.

Shock treatment

The third type of correction is an electric shock that the dog receives whenever he barks. The same training philosophy applies, but this collar gives an arguably more disagreeable correction.

Which works best?

Of the many dog owners that I have queried over the years, the majority said that electric shock bark collars are the most effective. However, most people (myself included) are not too thrilled with the prospect of shocking their dog. As a result, the other two bark collars are more commonly used. Many people have had great success with the citronella collars, which are a relatively new innovation.

More Tips for Preventing Barking

You may be able to calm a barker with a variety of small steps. Give these a try, as one or more of them may help. You should also read about separation anxiety (Chapter 13) if you suspect this is contributing to your adopted dog's barking problem when you're not home.

* Do not isolate your dog in a backyard run, basement, garage, or other area that is removed from your living space, even when you are not home. Most dogs, and especially adopted dogs, are very attuned to signs of being excluded or abandoned. Your job is to build security and trust, not undermine it.

* Leave a radio or television on low when you go out. Experiment with talk shows, classic music, jazz, popular tunes, news, etc. Who knows what your dog likes?

* Close windows and shades that face the street. Pedestrians and traffic, especially if they are close to the house or apartment, may constantly stimulate a dog to bark.

* Try leaving an unwashed T-shirt or other not too valuable item of clothing on your dog's bed. Your scent may provide security to a nervous dog.

* Exercise your dog. A tired dog will be more likely to curl up and go to sleep than run around barking.

* Practice short absences from home, building up to longer times away. However, no dog should be alone for more than half a day without a bathroom break, exercise, and companionship.

* Adopt another dog. Companionship may quiet your barker. It is possible, though, that you'll end up with two dogs that bark! Choose a basenji—a dog that does not bark—if you want to take no chances.

But barking is normal!

Two decades ago when I was first exposed to bark collars, I had much trepidation about them for a couple of reasons. At the time, the only type of collar available was the shock variety. I personally hate getting electric shocks, and I don't like the idea of shocking dogs, either.

Then along came shock corrections with yard containment systems, such as Invisible Fence. I have come to accept these systems. Why? A few shocks are certainly preferable to being run over by a school bus or poisoned by radiator fluid or lost in the next county—all the potential dangers facing a roaming dog. An unpleasant correction for trying to leave the backyard is not a terrible alternative to disaster.

With an excessive barker, shock corrections may be better than eviction from an apartment, being fined for breaking local noise ordinances, and disturbing household members or neighbors who cannot tolerate the noise.

Also, I was understandably concerned about the basic premise of bark collars. Barking is normal for dogs! Preventing it altogether is wrong. I worried that a dog that becomes fearful of *ever* barking might experience some adverse backlash effects. Most dogs need to bark sometimes—simply because they are dogs.

Have no fear

My fears were put to rest as I talked with dog owners and trainers that had lots of experience with the bark collar. Without exception, everyone said essentially the same thing: "Oh no, she's not afraid to bark. She knows when that collar is on and when it is off. When the collar's on, she doesn't make a peep. But when the collar's not on she still barks her fool head off. We only use the bark collar when we need her to be quiet."

Personally, I have never used a bark collar with one of my own dogs. It is no longer because I have a problem with the correction they give. I am not one of these trainers that have a confused bias toward the use of negative reinforcement when used properly in training. I have just never been in a situation where the Quiet command was not sufficient with my dogs. That is why I have collected feedback for many years from pet owners and trainers who have needed to rely on these devices.

If Quiet on Command training does not work quickly with your dog, or you need a noisy dog to be quiet when you are not at home, certainly give a bark training collar a try. I will make a few important suggestions. Get an experienced trainer's help. The clerk in the pet supply shop who sells you the device is not my definition of an experienced trainer. At the very least, study the owner's manual carefully and follow the training and safety tips in it. If you can control the intensity of the collar's correction, start low. Increase it only if you are using the collar correctly and it is not effective.

Use the collar only part-time, not twenty-four hours a day. Again, dogs need to bark; I believe it is emotionally harmful to silence them forever. As our beloved pets, they have a right to communicate. Making your world a little quieter is certainly reasonable, but it would be a sadder and less safe world without a dog's bark. Use a bark training collar wisely.

Chapter 12

Problems with Food

FOR MANY DOGS, feeding time is the high point of their day. They may eat their food in one sitting or nibble at it throughout the day. While the dog is eating, family members can walk by or pick up the dish or stroke the dog's back. If someone offers a tidbit of human food, the dog can take it gently without mauling fingers or hands.

For other dogs, food is the trigger for some nightmarish behavior. Aggression around food is a serious problem, especially when children are in the home. Food gobbling, finicky eating, and food stealing also cause problems for owners. If your adopted dog has any of these issues with food, this chapter will give you some practical advice for improving his behavior.

Guarding the Food Bowl

One reason that some dogs are given away and end up in shelters is that they are aggressive toward people or other pets that get near their food bowl. For the most part, these dogs often have perfectly good dispositions under all other circumstances. Food seems to make them crazy.

I have met individuals that change so dramatically while eating that it is astounding. Their Jekyll and Hyde personalities are both baffling and upsetting to their owners. For some reason, either known or unknown, these dogs feel seriously threatened while eating. They respond to that threatening feeling with varying degrees of aggression.

Fight fire with fire?

Early in my dog-training career I was taught that the best way to handle food-bowl aggression was with counteraggression toward the dog. Older trainers advised me to "get tough and shake him down." That was the approach most commonly used a few decades ago.

Although the "get tough" method occasionally worked, it often failed miserably. In most cases this approach only made the dog's behavior worse. Over the years I have found a better way that works with many dogs. Look at it as a simple mathematical equation.

Divide dog's kibble: add food, subtract aggression

Start by dividing your dog's meal into eight parts. Place the empty food bowl on the floor. When your dog goes to the bowl, add a portion of kibble. When he is almost done, add the next portion. Continue to add food to the bowl until the food is gone.

As you do this technique, praise your dog, using a quiet, soothing tone of voice—as long as the dog is not growling while he eats. If he does growl, say "Nhaa!" in a guttural tone and stop adding food. When he stops growling, add another portion of kibble.

No magic solution

You may have to repeat this technique for several weeks or more before this problem dissipates. Initially, only one person should do this procedure. This person should be an adult. *Children should never be expected to handle aggression problems.* In fact, keep small children away from the food bowl altogether. Keep other pets and people away from the dog specifically during mealtimes. More than one person hovering around the eating area will only make the dog feel more threatened. Your goal is to take apprehension away. After a couple of weeks, if the dog is doing well, other adult family members can try this procedure.

A word of caution: This is a great technique to try on dogs that are mildly protective of their food. If your adopted dog is seriously aggressive around food, perhaps attacking or biting anyone that simply comes near at feeding time, do not use this technique. You have a much bigger problem than "food issues." As I have said before in this book, a dangerously aggressive dog does not belong in a pet home. See Chapter 10, "Mouthing and Biting Problems," and Chapter 16, "When the Best Efforts Fail," for help in assessing your problem.

Multiple Dogs

The best thing you can do if your dog is food-aggressive toward other dogs in the household is to alter the mealtime environment. Specifically, feed multiple dogs separately. Put up baby gates or close doors to keep them apart while they eat. Or feed one outside (in a fenced area, of course) and one inside. Or put them all outside, and bring them inside, one at a time, to eat.

When I lived with three adult male dogs, they all ate at the same time but at opposite corners of my kitchen. I stood in the middle supervising. The Labs finished first (surprise, surprise) but could not cross the room to another's food bowl without a "Nhaa!" correction from me. They all learned to wait in their respective corners until the last eater was finished. Then it was an enthusiastic three-dog switch, as they all checked out each other's empty bowls for stray crumbs.

Protecting food from subordinate pack members is a natural canine behavior. Even dogs that get along wonderfully, as my three males did, may get testy with each other when it comes to their food. Again, the best way to avoid possible fights is to give each dog his own eating space. Do whatever is necessary to enforce that space.

On the other hand, protecting food from human family members is not acceptable behavior. Your dog must not be allowed to view you as a pack subordinate. The technique of adding food to your dog's bowl, described above, reinforces your pack-leader image. That's because when they are so inclined, pack leaders share food with subordinates. Your dog may not tolerate other dogs near his dish, but he has to learn to tolerate you.

Food Gobbling

Food gobbling is not a behavior problem that sends dogs to the shelter. But it is annoying and can create digestion problems. Dogs that "wolf down" their food can easily choke. Often they also throw up the food minutes after they have finished eating. Fortunately, this behavior does not cause dogs to become too thin, because most dogs are not at all reluctant to re-eat the vomit. (Disgusting to us, I admit.) But who wants to clean up the mess, especially when it appears on a rug or other absorbent surface? Probably no one, especially on a frequent basis.

In dogs with shortened faces, such as bulldogs and pugs, food gobbling can even interfere with breathing. I'll never forget the sad phone call I received from a client whose French bulldog had died earlier that day after aspirating its food.

Many dogs learn to gobble food while living in a kennel setting. Your adopted dog may come to you with this habit. Shelter workers normally feed all of the shelter dogs at about the same time, and group feeding creates competition. Even though the dogs are kenneled separately, they can see, hear, and smell the other dogs eating. The mind-set becomes "Eat as fast as you can before the guy next door gets it!"

Food-gobbling behavior is not created solely in dog shelters. It is also common in multiple-dog households. Many dogs, even ones that have come from good breeders, eat like this, as my three males did. Eating as much as possible as fast as possible is a natural canine behavior. In the wild, wolves do not know when their next meal is coming. They also know that a pack member or a scavenging animal will take their food if given the chance. So eating quickly and gorging on food is necessary for survival in the wild.

Your adopted dog lives in a domestic situation, of course, where all needs are met every day. If you find the dog's food gobbling to be a problem, here are two things to try.

One solution: spread it around

Find an area away from other dogs and dump your dog's bowl of kibble on the floor. The dog will have to pick up the kibble one or two pieces at a time. This technique is a great way to slow down eating. Yes, it's a little messy. However, dogs that are enthusiastic eaters do a thorough job of cleaning up.

Some owners have told me that they even dump their dog's dry food on the lawn. This makes the dog's cleanup even more methodical. Some say that this lawn technique helps the dog fulfill his hunting instinct. I do know that zookeepers now use a similar technique with some types of zoo animals. "Hunting" through the habitat for food tidbits engages the animal's natural instincts and behaviors. It also provides mental stimulation to the captive creatures.

Another solution: eating around an obstacle

Another technique that you can try is placing an obstacle, such as a tennis ball or rubber "Kong" toy, in the dog's food bowl. Working around the object to get to each piece of kibble takes time. It helps slow down eating.

A word of caution: Dog geniuses may foil this plan. I have had some owners report to me that their smart dogs would remove the obstacle object from the bowl—and then proceed to gobble their food. One owner told me that her black Labrador was simply so ravenous that the tennis ball would just get knocked out of the bowl during his feeding frenzy. She did ask me in a very concerned voice, "There's no chance that he will eat the ball, is there?" I guess with hungry Labs you never know.

Food Stealing

People are often amazed and baffled when their dogs steal food. Owners will ask me, "Why does he do this? We feed him twice a day, and he gets plenty of treats." The answer is easy: Canines are scavengers.

While it is true that wolves and coyotes are predators that hunt for their food, their diet is often supplemented by scavenging. Carcasses that have been left by other predators can be a source of food. Campsites that are abandoned or left unattended may be raided. Garbage cans or dump areas are easy pickings. Even fresh road kill can help fill a hungry canine's belly.

Domestic dogs, like their wild canine cousins, are also great opportunists. To most dogs there is no such thing as too much food. Your adopted dog may be strongly prone to stealing food, especially if he was a street waif or habitual wanderer.

My late Australian shepherd, Drifter, was an extraordinary food thief, even though I got him as a young puppy. On one memorable day when Drifter was about five years old, he tipped over our large plastic dog-food container. I had been out sailing for an hour or so. When I

Food-Obsessed!

Some dogs seem to think about nothing but food, even when they are healthy and well fed. They may whine whenever you are eating. They may bark to demand their dinner. They may steal food at every opportunity. If this describes your adopted dog, don't despair. Now is a great time to put obedience skills to work.

* Whining and barking: The Quiet on Command exercise usually solves whining and barking problems. See Chapter 11 for specific training steps. Also, be careful not to reinforce whining or barking by giving the dog a tidbit of food "to shut him up." You actually are making this bad habit even stronger.

* Begging at the table: Down-Stay is your solution. A dog cannot lie down and stay and beg at the same time. Practice this exercise every day for best results. See Chapter 23.

* Food stealing: Tighten the ship! Clear off tabletops and counters; buy a trash can with a lid; put groceries away promptly. And, of course, supervise your dog. Baby gates can keep a dog out of the kitchen or dining room, either permanently or during mealtimes.

got back to the house, I found Drifter munching away. I had just filled the container that morning with forty pounds of kibble, and much of it was gone. He looked as if he had swallowed a basketball!

I called my veterinarian, who had me immediately bring him in for an exam. He kept Drifter for observation for several hours. Before I brought him home, I was instructed not to let him drink too much water—just little sips throughout the night. I did not feed that food-thieving mutt a full meal for three days.

Drifter stole lots of food in his fourteen years. He trained Barbara and me to make sure that all food was put out of his reach whenever he was left alone. We had to learn to be craftier than the dog, and occasionally we failed. He enjoyed steak, an entire birthday cake, bagels, and grilled fish, to name just a few foods. Unfortunately, Drifter passed down his scavenging prowess to my puppy, Crea. Crea is now eight years old and has successfully stolen her share of food.

Two styles of food thievery

Almost all dogs will steal food if given the opportunity. An untrained dog with food-thief tendencies may brazenly get up on a kitchen counter and grab food right in front of his owner. He might even have the nerve to steal your pork chop right off your dinner plate while you sit at the table.

A well-trained dog with these same tendencies would never behave this way. He's craftier! He will wait until you are not paying attention to strike. This was how Drifter and Crea operated. Given the chance, they always loved to steal food. And they were always aware when a chance came along.

A well-trained food thief

You need well-timed corrections in order to train a dog not to take food off the table right in front of you. As in any other training, corrections that come after the fact are ineffective and do nothing but confuse the dog.

The best time to correct your dog for food stealing is when you feel he is thinking about it. When your dog looks at the bread on the table or kitchen counter, look him in his face and growl "Nhaa!" To further reinforce your authority, make the dog do a Down-Stay for five or ten minutes. It sends a follow-up message that you are in control.

The next-best time to correct your dog for food stealing is just as he makes his move for the food. After he has grabbed the bread and gulped it down, it's too late. With well-timed corrections, your dog will respect you as pack leader and never grab food—as long as the pack leader is paying attention.

Can I train my dog to never steal food?

With some dogs the answer is yes. However, I don't really have a specific technique, because it depends a lot on the dog. In theory, if you left the room and something disagreeable happened to your dog precisely as he was snatching food, he would learn to avoid snatching food—or at least that particular kind of food. The problem is, how do you do it? Surveillance cameras, motion detectors, and remote-control shock collars might work. But that is highly impractical for most pet owners. Your own surveillance and vigilance are the keys to success.

A positive training approach?

One of the goofiest things I heard about recently was a trainer's claim that she only used "positive training" methods. She was quoted as saying that she never punished dogs for any misdeeds. If her dogs did an undesirable behavior, she simply told them, "Too bad, no cookie!"

I would love to see how well "Too bad, no cookie!" works as your eighty-five-pound golden retriever is ingesting your filet mignon. All I can say is, beware of such nonsense. A corrective "Nhaa!" is certainly appropriate for undoing problem behaviors. Don't be afraid to use it.

Snack-Snatching

Almost all dogs love snacks. It's pleasurable for us owners to give out doggie treats or a tidbit of our own food. It's *not* pleasurable to have our fingers practically bitten off by a food grabber.

Every dog, adopted or not, should learn to take a treat gently from his owner's hand. All you need to teach it is a firm grip on the treat and a good growl ("Nhaa!"). Here's what to do.

Have your dog sit on command and stay. If he has not learned this yet, clip the leash to his collar. Hold the leash near the clip—close enough so that he cannot jump up at your hand or face. Hold the treat in your other hand and show it to him. If he gets wild, put the treat away and correct him with a firm growl—"Nhaa!" Remember, you are the pack leader. You can hold food without your dog jumping all over you.

When your dog remains sitting, give the command "Easy" and move the treat slowly toward his mouth. The moment he lunges for it or tries to grab it from your hand, pull your hand back and growl "Nhaa!" Say "Easy" and try again.

I have sometimes moved a treat toward and away from a dog's mouth about a dozen times until he has managed a gentle mouth. With well-timed corrections and the withdrawal of the treat, the dog eventually understands what he must do to get it. You should break one dog biscuit into several small pieces so that you can practice more than once each time you give out a treat.

One training session won't forever banish a dog's treat-grabbing behavior. Even my eight-year-old springer spaniel, Crea, needs a refresher session once in a while. But I do try to prevent grabbing each and every time she gets a treat by saying "Easy" as I give it to her. She has learned this command through the training described here, and she is usually very good at obeying it.

This training has proved especially helpful for my young daughter. She can tell Crea, "Easy!" and give her a dog cookie or other treat without harm. It has helped our child to enjoy our family dog and not be afraid to hand her food.

Finicky Eaters

Dogs that have no competition for food—or are overly indulged with food—sometimes become spoiled and become fussy eaters. This is usually more distressing to owners than it is harmful to the dogs. These dogs are confident that food will always be available, so they are not compelled to eat more than they really need. Put out fresh food each day. Unless ill, a dog will not starve himself to death.

If your dog is terribly thin, you can try techniques such as wetting dry kibble with a little warm water to make a gravy. Experience shows that dogs will eat more when dry kibble has water added to it. Adding a wet canned-meat dog food also will increase taste appeal and encourage dogs to eat more.

It is possible that your dog is turning up his nose at the food you offer because it is rancid. His nose knows! This is especially true with foods not containing preservatives. At the very least, replace the food he is reluctant to eat with a fresh bag. Check the expiration date to be sure.

If you know that your adopted dog was a good eater before he came to you, you may want to find out what brand of food he ate. Use it for a few weeks or months. It is a small adjustment for you, but it may be an important familiar comfort to your adopted dog. As long as he came from a caring environment, your dog may find reassurance in eating the familiar food. On the other hand, if you are rescuing your dog from abuse, I would recommend intentionally *changing* the food he once ate (if you know what it was). This is one of many subtle ways to show an adopted dog that his old life is over and that a new life is beginning.

Dogs That Have Suffered Neglect

Some adopted dogs were actually starved by their previous owners. They may have been left tied in a backyard, locked in a basement, or confined somewhere else. Little or no food may have been provided to them for weeks on end.

Dogs that have suffered this kind of abuse need medical evaluation and a nutritional rehabilitation plan. You definitely need the guidance of a good veterinarian. He or she will help you develop a feeding regime that can, I hope, restore your adopted dog to health.

A dog of this description certainly may have behavioral problems around food in addition to medical concerns. Generally speaking, take care of the medical problems first. As your dog's physical health and emotional well-being are restored, you can turn your attention to improving his food-related behavior.

Chapter 13

Separation Anxiety

THIS IS THE BIGGEST PROBLEM that some adopted dogs face. These dogs are acutely aware of being abandoned once by their previous owners, maybe more than once if several owners were involved. Now, for all they know, it may happen again.

Dogs that suffer from separation anxiety may bark excessively, chew forbidden items, dig up the yard, lick themselves until wounds appear, urinate or defecate indoors, etc. These are dogs that cannot relax and behave appropriately when left alone, and as a result they have some very unhappy owners.

What causes separation anxiety? The roots of it sometimes lie in early puppyhood, if the pup was taken from its mother at too young an age. More often it is caused by abandonment, which all adopted dogs have experienced to some degree. Consider the very nature of dogs. It will give you a much better understanding of this difficult problem.

A wolf in dog's clothing

In the wild, canines that live in packs are rarely alone. Each individual in the pack has a role that benefits all the pack members. Some go off to hunt together. Others stay behind to watch over puppies or to guard the den area. Regardless of his or her specific job, each individual is almost always with other pack members.

Whenever pack members reunite, they instinctively greet one another. For puppies, the return to the den of adult pack members is a joyous occasion. Puppies greet returning adults by excitedly running up to them with tails submissively wagging. Adults nuzzle, lick, and play with them. If a hunt was successful, the adults regurgitate food for the puppies. For these social canines, togetherness is important for adults and puppies alike.

Like wolves, domestic dogs are pack animals. They are wired in many of the same ways as their wild cousins. Instinctively, domestic dogs also expect to be with members of their pack all of the time. When a domestic puppy is born, he is part of a pack right from the beginning—his litter. He has brothers, sisters, and a mother dog that are with him at all times. The breeder and his or her family and friends visit and regularly handle the puppies. Each puppy becomes socialized with humans, whom I believe they view as part of the extended pack.

How to create separation anxiety

At around eight weeks old, the puppy is sold or given to a new home. If he has been properly socialized during the first weeks of his life, the transition from the puppy pack into his new human pack is smooth. The puppy enthusiastically interacts with each family member and quickly bonds with them.

One day everybody leaves. The kids go off to school, for example, and Mom and Dad leave for work. They will be back, but the puppy does not know this. All he knows is that his pack has abandoned him.

Naturally he feels stressed and anxious. In an attempt to release this stress, the puppy begins to bark and howl. This gets no results. The pack has not come back for him and he is still alone.

He tries digging at the door through which the pack left. Maybe he can get out and find them. When this does not work, he gets frustrated and chews and rips to shreds anything in the room. Newspapers, shoes, sofa cushions, it doesn't matter. Chewing helps alleviate some of the stress and frustration that he is feeling.

Several hours later the pack returns. To the puppy, their absence may have felt like eternity. He believed that they were gone for good. But at least the pack has returned. Unfortunately, the relief and joy that he feels is short-lived.

When one of the human pack members walks into the house, he or she sees the scratched door and chewed household items. Tempers flare. "You bad puppy! You stupid dog! Look what you did!" shouts the owner. Even worse, some puppies are physically disciplined.

Now the puppy is really emotionally shaken up. After a stressful day of feeling abandoned by the pack, the puppy's situation has taken a turn for the worse. The pack has miraculously returned, but he is treated like an intruder. No one greets him or acts happy that they are together again. What could this mean?

The next day the pack leaves again, and the previous day's chain of events is repeated. The owners have no idea why the puppy is behaving this way. They must have gotten a bad puppy, they think. Or the puppy is just mad about being left behind, and he's "getting even."

The puppy is totally confused, too. He feels extremely anxious about being left alone. It is not natural. He also is wondering if the day will come when the pack does not return. When they do come back each day, they are angry. The puppy seems to be the pack scapegoat.

After a few months

Puppies instinctively want to be a valued member of their pack. As the puppy is growing bigger, he will try to move up the pack hierarchy ladder. He will use behaviors that he learned with his littermates to improve his social ranking in this new pack.

Biting, growling, and jumping seem to work well. These behaviors make the adult female and the two adolescents squeal and act submissively toward him. Maybe if he can dominate them he will be treated with more respect within the pack! He has learned it is best to avoid the adult male and not to try these behaviors with him.

By the time the puppy is an adolescent, the patterns described here have been repeated many times. Destructive behavior around the house has become a daily routine. When the family returns home each day, items have been destroyed, and the dog is yelled at. In general, the dog is no fun for this family. He chews their personal possessions. He jumps up, he bites, and he does not listen. This dog has not worked out. Time to get rid of him.

Dad takes the dog to the shelter, where he is dropped off. Through the human perspective, a nuisance has been eradicated. Through the dog's point of view, *his daily fears of abandonment by his pack have been fulfilled.*

A Second Chance

Many, many dogs fit the profile described above. They are destroyed at shelters and pounds by the thousands year after year. Fortunately, people who want to give a dog a second chance save some dogs from this fate. However, when people do adopt one of these dogs, they risk taking on an individual with emotional baggage. It is the baggage of separation anxiety.

Separation anxiety manifests itself in various ways. The experience of being given away can cause lifelong problems in some dogs. With other dogs the damage is not so pronounced. Human beings have different personalities, too. Three different people robbed at gunpoint may have three different reactions to this upsetting experience.

It is the same with dogs. Abandonment can be so traumatic for some dogs that they never learn to be confident when left alone again. The very worst thing that can happen to such a dog is to be abandoned multiple times. Separation anxiety could be at the root of your dog's problem behaviors if he has experienced several adoptions.

Fortunately, most dogs that have been abandoned—if they are handled properly—can learn to feel secure when their pack leaves the house. They can learn to behave themselves when alone, confident that the pack will soon reunite joyfully.

No dog likes to be left alone

I have never owned a dog that was happy about being left alone. I think my dog's very favorite words are "Do you want to go?" Most dog owners would probably agree that their dogs feel the same way.

Because of good handling, I never had a puppy whose anxiety about being alone developed into a behavioral problem. I conditioned my puppies to curl up and go to sleep or to chew on appropriate doggie toys when I left the house. They stayed out of trouble, so my return home was always a joyful one. We were both happy to see each other, which built my puppy's confidence about enduring my absence. By the time the puppy was an adult, he knew the routine and could be well behaved and calm until I returned.

You can accomplish the same thing with an older dog that you adopt. The techniques described here will help your adopted dog adjust to short-term separation and to behave appropriately in your absence.

A structured environment

If your newly adopted dog shows any signs of separation anxiety, you cannot give him freedom in the house when you leave. Doing so will only give the dog an opportunity to repeat over and over again his problem behaviors. You must enforce proper behavior in your home right from the beginning.

To do this, you need to provide your dog with a structured environment when he is left alone. This environment must be safe, secure, and free of items that are inappropriate to chew. In this environment your dog will have two basic options: curl up and go to sleep or chew on his own toys.

A doggie condo

I use a kennel crate with my dogs. Depending on the dog, a blocked-off laundry room or kitchen might work just as well, although some dogs may be able to escape from these areas. Others might chew woodwork, curtains, linoleum, throw rugs, etc. Kennel crates are not easy to escape from, and there is nothing inside inappropriate to chew.

Whenever you leave your dog, place him in his structured environment. Provide him with doggie chew toys. Keep in mind that chewing helps dogs to release anxiety and frustration. The act of chewing is not the problem, it's chewing your household items.

Medical Intervention

A word of wisdom: If these methods do not help at all and your dog's separation anxiety only seems to be getting worse, consult your veterinarian. I have known owners with dogs that practically had panic attacks when left alone, even for just a few minutes. One large dog habitually broke through windows and screens whenever his owners left the house. The owners came to fear for their dog's safety.

A veterinarian can prescribe medication for a dog that seems to lose emotional control, despite good handling and a caring environment. Behavior-altering drugs can be useful in such situations. As a last resort, they may be the difference between keeping a dog and giving him up, again, for adoption.

Short and sweet

It is important that you start off by leaving your adopted dog for short periods only. Walk outside to chat with a neighbor, or go for a ride around the block. When you return, greet your dog joyfully and give him a small dog treat. Short trips will allow you to reinforce often that you are always coming back. A doggie treat when you return will fulfill your dog's primal instinct that the hunters are sharing the kill with valued pack members back at the den.

Over time, gradually increase the time that you leave your dog. Go from a half hour to a full hour. Never leave your dog crated for more than four hours at a time. If you work full-time, make arrangements that allow you to come home to take your dog out and spend some time with him. If this is not possible, enlist the help of a friend or neighbor. There are also pet care services that you can hire for this purpose.

How long?

With lots of repetition and consistency, your adopted dog will build a habit of good behavior in your absence. He will grow confident that you will always return. Because of the structured environment, he will curl up and go to sleep or chew on his own toys while you are gone. He will *not* be practicing destructive behaviors, such as chewing up the house. As a result, your reunion will always be a positive one, providing your dog with further reassurance about enduring your absence.

The goal of most pet owners is to have their dog loose in the house while they are gone. My dogs have this freedom, but only because they do not get into trouble. I used a kennel crate to teach this skill to every one of my dogs, no matter what their age. Even Jossie, the problem-filled adopted poodle described in Chapter 24, learned to behave when I went out.

How long will this take with your dog? Truthfully, it is not possible to set up a timetable for any dog-training objective. Dogs learn and form habits at a different rate. What takes one dog a few weeks to learn may take another dog several months. Puppies are a bit easier to predict than older dogs. An adolescent adopted dog with only a few separation problems can reasonably be expected to overcome them faster than a middle-age dog with some deep-seated bad habits.

A good rule of thumb for any timetable estimates is what I call the "equal time" rule. You must give at least as much time to repeating a new behavior as the old behavior existed. In other words, if a dog has been chewing inappropriate items for a year, then it will take a year to break the habit.

But persevere. With consistency and practice, your dog's behavior will only get better. In your caring hands his fears of abandonment and his problem behaviors will become a distant memory for both of you.

Chapter 14

Shy and Submissive Dogs

IF YOUR ADOPTED DOG has either of these personality traits—or both of them—you face certain challenges that other dog owners do not. Fortunately, most problems relating to shyness or submissiveness can be successfully managed. If you handle these issues right, there is no reason for them to undo your adoption success.

Why are dogs shy?

Dogs are shy basically for two reasons. They either have a genetic disposition to shyness or they were not properly socialized.

A dog with an innately spooky or "flighty" personality will, in all likelihood, have puppies with a similar personality. This shy personality trait is prevalent in some specific breeds, such as the Shetland sheepdog, German shepherd, and Chihuahua. From a handling perspective, owners of innately shy dogs should use the same techniques as for dogs that were poorly socialized (described below). The training goal is the same: a stable, obedient, and more confident dog.

Improper socialization

Dogs that were never socialized—or received improper socialization— often turn out shy. Why? Exposure to people, places, and things in the early stages of puppyhood is essential to personality development. It helps to create confident, outgoing adult dogs.

Timing is important, too. During development, a puppy has several fear-imprint periods. Traumatic experiences during these periods can stay with a puppy throughout life. For example, let's say that a bearded man wearing a baseball cap accidentally stepped on a puppy's foot. It caused the pup to yip in pain. After a short time the puppy would probably get over it. However, if this same experience happened during a fear-imprint period, the puppy could develop a lifetime fear of bearded men wearing baseball caps.

Knowledgeable dog breeders are aware of fear-imprint periods in the first weeks and months of a dog's life. Good breeders are careful to protect their puppies from bad experiences during these times.

A bad experience during a fear-imprint period is not the only way to create shyness. Just being sequestered away from the sights and sounds of the world can cause this problem. Although dog owners must be careful not to let young puppies have traumatic experiences, it is equally important that they allow their puppies and adolescents to "get out in the world." It is an essential ingredient for raising a confident adult dog.

The Right Home for a Shy Dog

Adoptable dogs with shy personalities are often difficult to place. When potential owners walk through an animal shelter checking out dogs, they are not drawn to the aloof dog in the back of the cage or the quivering pup with fear in his eyes. The gregarious dog that comes up to the door, wagging his tail and looking cute, is naturally the one to attract a lot of positive attention.

One appealing feature of shy dogs is that they are extremely devoted to their owners. And just because a dog is shy does not mean that he is not smart or trainable. However, a shy dog is not the right fit for every household.

Shy dogs do well in quiet, controlled environments. This usually means an adult home. A busy home with children often proves too overwhelming for a shy dog. Kids and their friends plus parents on the run—this kind of household tends to keep the fearful dog in a perpetual state of angst.

A person who lives alone or a couple without children can provide a shy dog a home where stress is minimal. Fortunately, people-shy dogs are not ordinarily frightened of other dogs. The household of a single person or couple without children can usually enjoy multiple dogs—even multiple shy dogs—without a problem.

Fear Biters

Some dogs are so scared of people that they become fear biters. Fortunately, most dogs first opt to escape from situations that frighten them rather than to bite. But without escape as an option, some of these dogs will panic and bite. This often happens when fearful dogs are on a leash. A person bends over to pet the dog, and snap! That's why I counsel everyone, especially children, to ask the owner before greeting a strange dog. If in doubt, don't reach out. Just a friendly "Hi, pup!" will do.

It goes without saying: Never back a scared dog into a corner, even if the dog knows you. His instinct to protect himself from a perceived threat will probably mean a painful bite for you.

Fearful dogs often show their teeth and growl before launching an attack. But this is not always true. Even without a pre-strike warning, a trained eye can see signs that a frightened dog will snap or bite. The dog's entire body becomes stiff. The hair on the top of his shoulders stands up. The dog's tail may be wrapped tightly between his legs. And the eyes will flicker. This flicker may be subtle, but it will be there. If this dog has no way to get away, he probably will bite.

A Case Study: Jena, the Shy Shorthair

One of the first dogs that I owned was Jena, a German shorthaired pointer. I adopted her when she was six months old. There had been nine puppies in Jena's litter. Seven of them were sold at eight weeks old. The breeder kept for himself two puppies that he believed had great bird-hunting potential.

This man had raised and hunted over German shorthairs for many years. When Jena's litter was born, he was in his late eighties. By the time his two pups had turned six months old, he concluded that his health was too poor for the task of training these dogs. He decided to place the two pups with someone who would bird-hunt with them. That's how I came into the picture.

"Don't Look at the Tail, Boy"

The smartest dog trainer that I ever knew was an eighty-two-year-old beagle trainer from Mississippi. This gentleman may have had only a third-grade education in the world of academics, but he had a master's degree in the world of dogs.

This beagle man was a good friend of a veterinarian that I once worked for. He used to hang out at the veterinary office periodically and brighten our days with tales of bunny hunting with a pack of hounds.

One day the beagle man accompanied me into the kennel. I was getting a shy Doberman-shepherd mix that needed sutures removed. This dog had a spooky personality and would growl fearfully whenever anyone stopped by her kennel cage to talk to her.

I had made some progress at making friends with her. After her first day in the hospital, she had stopped growling at me when I squatted by her cage and told her that she was a good girl. On that particular morning, I opened her cage door to find her with raised gums, showing her teeth and growling. But the odd thing was, she was wagging her tail a mile a minute.

I was very hesitant, not knowing what to do. I asked myself, should I reach in and try to loop the leash over her head, or was she going to try to bite me?

The beagle trainer stood several feet away watching. Finally I looked at him and verbalized what had been going on in my mind. "She's growling, but her tail is wagging. Do you think she will bite?"

His response: "Don't look at the tail, boy. That ain't the end that bites!"

I learned that day that dogs sometimes wag their tails when they are extremely anxious. Although a wagging tail often means a happy dog, it can also mean the exact opposite. Keep your eyes on the end with the teeth!

Love at first sight?

When I first met Jena, she would not come near me. She only seemed to care about the breeder. When I approached, she cowered and hung her head. I looked at the breeder and said, "I don't know about her. I don't think she likes me."

He said, "Oh no, don't worry, she will be fine. Trust me. I know my dogs. Take her home and give her a few days to get to know you. If you don't like her by the end of the week, bring her back. I'll return your money."

Live and learn

By the end of the first week, Jena still would not come anywhere near me. If I approached her, she would hang her head and act as if I were going to beat her up! Let me be clear. The breeder had not physically abused Jena in any way. She was fine with him. She just acted afraid of me and anyone else who came into my house. Did I really want to keep a dog like this?

I was a dog rookie back then. The breeder was honest about our trial period and certainly would have given me my money back if I returned the dog. What I didn't know then was that I could not bring a puppy into my house for a week without becoming attached. Besides, if I was not going to love this shy misfit, who would?

Kennel shyness

As I started to research shyness in dogs, I learned that Jena was "kennel shy." Jena and her other littermate had lived in a small kennel in the breeder's backyard from the time that they were born. The mother dog lived in the house with the man and his wife.

The two pups had extremely limited human interaction during the first six months of their lives. The elderly breeder and his wife were the only people that the two dogs regularly interacted with. The breeder's house was in a fairly rural area, and the couple did not entertain many visitors.

I believe that the breeder loved his dogs and tried to do the best that he could with them under his circumstances. He fed the dogs twice a day and let them out into the yard to urinate and defecate several times a day. Once a day he practiced beginner hunting skills. He took each dog out of the kennel individually and played a game of fetch. He would throw a hard rubber retrieving dummy and, as the pup was racing after it, shoot a starter's pistol. Every day each dog got about twenty minutes of this game, which they loved. It was the high point of their day.

One inch at a time

I knew that if I was ever going to hunt birds and earn obedience titles with Jena, she would have to learn to trust me. And we would have to become friends. I used just about all of the techniques described in Chapter 8, "Bonding from Day One." These included long leash walks, extra food treats, and even some naps curled up together on the sofa. I also played fetch with her as the breeder had done. And I started communicating with her through obedience training.

Obedience Training: The Great Confidence Builder

I knew that Jena had to be a well-behaved dog to stay in my home. In fact, I had aspirations to earn obedience titles with her, as I had with my Irish setter, Jason. So I started taking her to a local dog obedience class once a week. What I did not realize was that obedience training would also build Jena's confidence.

Dogs are always most confident when they are doing something that is familiar to them. Obedience training gave Jena a whole repertoire of familiar, structured behaviors. For example, if I stopped on the street to chat with someone, Jena felt more secure and confident when she was told to sit and stay. Because she had a job to do—a simple Sit-Stay—shy Jena didn't fall apart around strangers. When a visitor came to my house, Jena acted much less nervous if she was told to lie down and stay. These are just two examples of the many ways in which obedience training made Jena feel and act more confident.

A valuable lesson about praise

On the first day of obedience class, I was talking to a woman about Jena. The woman was attempting to pet her, and Jena was straining on the leash to back away. I was using the leash to pull Jena toward the woman. As I did so, I was verbally reassuring her in a soothing tone: "It's okay, Jena. Nobody's going to hurt you. Good girl, it's okay."

All of a sudden the gruff obedience instructor came charging over. She looked me in the eye and said, "Stop praising that dog for acting shy! And never try to force a nervous dog on someone."

I said meekly, "I was just trying to reassure her."

"Well, you weren't. You were praising her."

I was intimidated and embarrassed. I never grew to appreciate this particular instructor's teaching style, but after thinking about what she said, I had to admit that she was right.

Anytime that a dog's behavior is rewarded with praise, food, petting, etc., that behavior is being reinforced. With enough reinforcement the behavior will become a habit. Jena could not understand that my comments were meant to reassure her and help her feel less nervous. She interpreted my soothing tones as praise for whatever she was doing at the time. Since she was shying away from someone, Jena thought her owner was praising her for shying away.

I learned to keep my mouth closed whenever Jena was acting shy. But I watched her closely. As soon as she showed any signs of relaxing, or better yet, made overtures of friendliness toward someone, I would quickly praise her.

My gruff instructor was also right about never trying to force a nervous dog on someone. I learned that doing so only makes a shy dog more reluctant to meet strangers.

Two long years

Building a shy dog's confidence is never a fast process. Patience is imperative. It is truly one inch at a time. It took two years of concentrated effort for Jena to no longer act like a basket case and become confident. During that two years I continued to do things with Jena to help her to love and trust me. I also practiced obedience exercises with her regularly. I did my best to try to expose Jena to the world by taking her with me whenever I could.

Jena never became an extrovert. I don't believe that most shy dogs ever will, even with excellent handling. But what Jena did do was become more stable and confident. That was enough for her to have a great life and become one of my all-time favorite dogs.

She also turned into a remarkable bird dog. We hunted pheasants together until she was ten years old. And she earned two American Kennel Club obedience titles. At one obedience trial, the judge remarked that Jena was a great heeling dog. I think that's because she wanted to stay as close to me—and as far away from the judge—as possible! She did heel beautifully and excelled in the other exercises, too. My Nervous Nellie earned a lot of high scores. She taught me that great dogs can come in shy packages. It just takes proper handling and a little patience to coax them out.

Sound Shyness

We tend to think that shyness means shyness of people. But some dogs have sound shyness. They are frightened by loud noises. In most cases, these dogs were improperly exposed to sound. They may have had firecrackers set off near them, or they were tied out near a trap shoot, or there was a booming thunderstorm during one of their fear-imprint periods. As a result, these dogs learned to fear loud noises. Even a single firing of a shotgun can scare dogs. Dogs must be in motion, doing something that they love, if they are going to make an agreeable association with the explosive sound of a shotgun.

It is much harder to undo sound shyness than it is to prevent it in the first place. If you can find ways to associate sound with food or other pleasurable activities, it may help your dog become less sensitive. At mealtime, try rattling a metal spoon around the inside of the metal food pan. Play a game of fetch with your dog whenever the lawn service shows up and turns on their noisy mowers. By distracting your dog with a fun activity, you can help him deal with some of his nervous-ness over sounds.

Dealing with thunder

Many dogs become anxious during thunderstorms. Interestingly, I have observed that as dogs become older, thunderstorms bother them more. I have known many dogs that were unfazed by thunderstorms in their early years and then started to act nervous as they reached middle age.

As with all shyness issues, owners must not inadvertently reinforce unwanted behavior. You may feel the urge to reassure your nervous dog during a thunderstorm with soothing words such as "Don't worry. You're safe. It's okay." Your dog is going to think that you are praising him for feeling the way he does. Say nothing to your dog during thunderstorms. Try to act as calmly and unfazed by the storm as possible.

Change the environment

You certainly can try to insulate your sound-shy dog from the noise of a storm. This will minimize his anxiety. Pull down window shades or close blinds. Put on music to muffle the sound of the thunder. If you are concerned about using electricity during a storm, buy a transistor radio.

If you are crate training or still have a crate because your dog enjoys it, kennel your dog during the storm. Many dogs like the secure feeling of their crate. You can place a sheet over the top and three sides of the crate so that the dog feels snug and safe in his den. Your dog's cousin the wolf probably crawls into a den during storms. Your crate can serve the same purpose—it is training through a canine point of view!

Our late yellow Labrador, Bentley, was sound-shy and hated thunderstorms. During a storm he was most content cuddled up next to Barbara on the sofa. She would sit and read, acting as though there was nothing to worry about. Bentley wasn't so sure, but Barbara's relaxed demeanor helped him to not overreact.

Some veterinarians recommend tranquilizers during thunderstorms. Unfortunately, storms often come up quickly. Because it takes at least a half hour for most sedatives to take effect, the storm has passed by the time the drug starts to work. All you end up with is a half-zonked-out dog for the next several hours. Nevertheless, you may want to discuss tranquilizers with your veterinarian if your dog is extremely anxious and other techniques are ineffective.

Object Shyness

Object shyness is more of a quirky personality trait than a behavioral problem. It is unlikely to influence an adoption's success, although I guess it is possible for a dog to be so neurotic about everyday objects that an owner could not live with him. I have never met a dog this extreme.

However, I have known and lived with object-shy dogs. They seem to fall into two categories. Some dogs are spooked by objects that are out of their normal context, while other dogs freak out over familiar, everyday objects, which they suddenly seem to notice for the first time in their lives. Here are two examples.

While pheasant hunting with my German shorthaired pointer, Jena, I came upon an old telephone pole sitting erect in the middle of a field. Jena stopped in her tracks, started snarling and growling, and slowly backed away, looking as though she was ready to bolt.

At first I thought a snake or some other animal was in the grass. But there wasn't. It was just the pole. I walked over and leaned against it. But Jena would not come near it. I tried to verbally coax her over, but doing so only made her seem more leery. A few months later she reacted the same way when we encountered a rusted fifty-five-gallon oil drum in the woods. Throughout her life Jena was always unnerved by normal objects that were not where she thought they should be.

In the late seventies I owned a bull mastiff for a short time. Cagney had several medical problems and only lived to be ten months old. The time I did spend with him was very rewarding, and to this day I'm very fond of the breed.

One day when Cagney was about seven months old, I heard this deep "Woof, woof, woof!" alarm barking coming from the downstairs bathroom. When I looked into the bathroom, I saw Cagney hunched down, the fur on his back standing straight up, tail tucked between his legs, barking like crazy at the toilet. Silly puppy!

I said nothing to him, having learned from my experiences with Jena that verbal coaxing only seems to make dogs worse. I simply sat on the toilet, grabbed a magazine, and acted as if everything was fine. After a few minutes Cagney inched his way over to me, sniffed the toilet, and started wagging his tail.

What to do about object shyness

There is nothing too dramatic to do. Just behave normally, as though everything is fine. Do not say anything. Verbal coaxing will be interpreted by your dog as praise for the way he is feeling and behaving. Soothing tones will only reinforce his fear response.

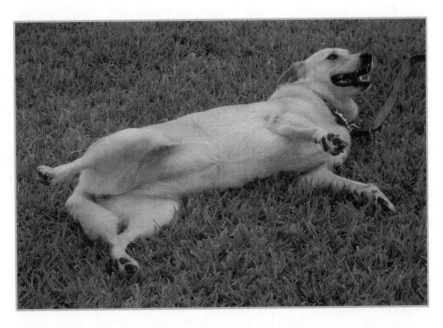

Dogs submit to a more dominant individual (human or canine) by rolling belly-up. Some extremely submissive dogs urinate when overwhelmed. This is not a housebreaking problem.

During adolescence many dogs go through a short phase when they react to normal everyday objects the way Cagney did. The majority of these pups outgrow this behavior. Reactions such as Jena's to out-of-context objects are probably caused by a lack of proper socialization early in the dog's life. Jena was object-shy all her life, but it wasn't a big problem.

Submissive Dogs

There are several basic traits that make up a dog's personality. We talked above about shy dogs. The opposite end of that spectrum is the dog that is a complete extrovert. These are the extremes. Most dogs fall somewhere in the middle on the shy-extrovert spectrum.

Another facet of dog personality is the submissive-versus-dominant spectrum. This trait is independent of a dog's gender, age, breed, or size. A dog of any description can be extremely dominant or extremely submissive. Fortunately, most dogs fall somewhere in the middle.

Submissive dogs should not be confused with shy dogs. There are many dogs with extroverted personalities that are very submissive, too.

The difference between dominant extroverts and submissive extroverts is evident in the way that they greet a person or another dog. The dominant extrovert will approach an individual with complete confidence. His shoulders will be up, his tail and ears held high. If this dog is an aggressive individual, be careful. He may charge straight ahead and even bite. An aggressive, dominant extrovert dog is not to be taken lightly.

On the other hand, a submissive extrovert will greet newcomers in a completely different way. She may run up to say hello, but ears, tail, and body posture will be low, maybe even slinky. When this individual reaches you, she may flop over, belly up. In some cases she will urinate (discussed below).

This dog's friendly but submissive behavior is often accompanied by a "submissive grin." The dog's lips are curled back with all her teeth showing. Sometimes the grin is accompanied with groans and moans.

The first time I observed a submissive grin was with my golden retriever, Woody, just after I got him. Woody was about a year and a

Is Your Dog Afraid of Dogs?

Some dogs are actually frightened of other dogs. This is especially true if they never interacted with other dogs before or they had a frightening dog experience somewhere in their past. Such an experience might make a dominant dog dog-aggressive (looking for fights for no apparent reason), but a submissive dog could easily react in just the opposite way, becoming fearful of all dogs.

If your adopted dog is dog-shy, you may only have a personality quirk on your hands, not a serious problem. Many dogs go through life without socializing with other dogs. As long as they get companionship from their human owners, family friends, and perhaps other pets, these dogs can be perfectly happy and well-behaved.

On the other hand, you may already own other dogs, have lots of dogs in your apartment building and neighborhood, and socialize with many dog-owning friends. Frequent dog contact is unavoidable.

My advice would be to try building your dog's confidence around other dogs. Find the sweetest, gentlest dog you know and allow the two dogs to spend some time together, preferably outdoors in a fenced area. Go on dog walks or off-leash dog hikes together. Practice obedience exercises in the same room. Make them both sit and stay, and then reward them both with a dog treat. These nonthreatening, enjoyable experiences will help a shy dog gain confidence.

As this chapter makes clear, you cannot expect to turn a shy dog into an outgoing extrovert. But you can bring about some changes and prevent the dog from "falling apart" in the presence of things that scare him.

half old when he came to live with me. Every time I came home Woody would greet me with a slinky body posture, his tail down low and flagging and his lips curled back. His teeth would be showing, and he would be grumbling.

I remember calling the breeder and saying, "What's with this dog?

When I come home he shows his teeth and growls!" She laughed, because she knew Woody well. "He's not growling," she said. "He's smiling at you and talking." She was right. Woody, my submissive extrovert, taught me about the submissive grin.

Submissive urination

Submissive urination often happens when extremely submissive dogs greet people and other dogs. For some dogs, peeing is just their natural response to the exciting yet intimidating moment of saying hello.

I get many letters from readers of my newspaper column, "Dog Talk," about dogs that do this. More often than not, the owners tell me that they are having a housebreaking problem. In fact, they are not. Submissive urination is unrelated to housebreaking. Dogs that are thoroughly trained to urinate and defecate outside can be submissive wetters. Yes, these dogs are urinating in the house, but they are not even aware that it is happening. Their submissive instinct kicks in, and their bladder simply lets go.

Will it go away?

Dogs of some breeds are more likely than others to experience submissive urination. These breeds include cocker spaniels, bichons, frises, poodles, golden retrievers, and Irish setters. Fortunately, most dogs that urinate submissively outgrow the behavior by the time they are a year old. However, some dogs never do. Among those that do not, a higher percentage are females.

It would not surprise me to know that many dogs are given away because of submissive urination. No one likes uncontrollable peeing in the house. But owners often do things that exacerbate this behavior. If you have adopted a dog that urinates submissively (especially if the dog is over a year old), you need to handle this individual properly. There is no reason for submissive urination to undo your adoption success.

First the bad news: There is no way to train a dog not to urinate submissively. Now the good news: Several techniques can help you manage this behavior and reduce its occurrence.

No corrections?

Do not correct your dog for urinating submissively in the house. Because dogs are not even aware that it is happening, they are not going to understand that they did something wrong. Even if they did understand why they are being corrected, they cannot control the behavior. It just happens. Correcting a dog for submissive urination is like correcting a dog for snoring. It's fruitless.

Actually, it's worse than fruitless. It's counterproductive. Corrections can be intimidating to submissive dogs, especially harsh corrections. Intimidating your submissive dog and making him nervous will only make his problem worse.

However, it is certainly okay to correct other unwanted behavior. Fortunately, your submissive dog will only need a mild correction for him to get the message. Overcorrections can easily cause a submissive dog to urinate. A simple, low-toned "Nhaa" will suffice in almost all situations.

Of course, no dog, regardless of his personality, should ever be over-corrected. However, a correction that is appropriate for a dominant dog will be an overcorrection for a submissive dog. It is important to temper your personality and handling skills to the personality of the dog you live with and train.

Another Case Study: Carrie, the Irish Setter

Carrie was my Irish setter Jason's mother. For many years after I got Jason, his dear sweet mom would stay with me when her owner was traveling. Carrie was a wonderful dog. She was beautiful and loving, with a long red coat and prematurely gray muzzle. But, boy, was she a submissive wetter. I would come home, and the tail would be wagging and the urine would be flying!

I discovered that the urinating did not begin until I spoke to Carrie. I quickly learned not to say a word or even *look* at her when I walked into the house. I would come in the front door and head right out the back door into the yard with the dogs following me. When I got the dogs on the grass, I would greet them all enthusiastically. Carrie would pee like a racehorse. She never outgrew her submissive urination, but I was able to minimize the mess. She was a welcome houseguest for many years.

Chapter 15

Overcoming the Scars of Abuse

Happily, most adopted dogs do not have a nightmarish past. Many are unclaimed strays that find new homes through a humane society. Some are turned in by their reasonably capable owners who could not (or would not) continue to care for them. Some are passed privately from one owner to another. Although these dogs may not have had the attention, training, and love that I believe all dogs deserve, they typically have been fed and housed and treated humanely most of their lives.

The truly unlucky dogs are those that were made to suffer at the hands of human beings. They may have been starved, chained outside, beaten, or worse. Females may have been subjected to bearing litter after litter of pups. Sick animals were never given medical care.

I have no sympathy or compassion for those who inflict pain and suffering on dogs. Case closed. Fortunately, I think we have become a more humane society than we were a hundred years ago, even a generation ago. Numerous laws now exist to protect animals from cruelty and abuse, and we willingly spend millions of dollars to meet our pets' nutritional, health, and behavioral needs. Yet I believe our society must continue to evolve—to a point where there is never any tolerance for neglect or mistreatment of any animals, whether it be dogs, cats, livestock, or wildlife. And it goes without saying that we must work harder to protect our children as well.

That said, some dogs do experience neglect and abuse. Somehow they survive what is inflicted on them and end up in an adopted home. If this is the case with your dog, first let me thank you. You are representing the good side of humanity to your pet and showing him that people are capable of kindness, not just causing pain. That is such a hopeful and important message! If you ever have a discouraging day with your dog, remind yourself that he may be learning for the first time what it's like to be loved and treated well. Your efforts are not in vain.

Advice from the Experts

Some dog professionals spend a lifetime handling and placing adopted dogs. They have a great deal of experience with identifying those dogs that can probably make it in a new home and those that are too dangerous or too ill to be somebody's pet. They make a lot of difficult decisions, and I admire their efforts.

Some of the dogs that these experts help get adopted are victims of abuse and neglect. The dogs find their way into adoption networks through all sorts of channels. Animal control officers rescue them, as strays they end up at the pound, sometimes relatives or neighbors intervene to save the dog. I've even heard of rescue workers buying or stealing abused dogs just to get them away from horrendous situations. After careful screening, many of these dogs, remarkably, are deemed capable of living with a new, loving family. Somehow they have survived with their health and good nature reasonably intact.

Which is not to say that they are unscathed. Dogs that have been abused or neglected may have all sorts of problems. Behavioral issues that are common to a large majority of untrained adolescent and adult dogs are described throughout this book. Some topics deserve special attention here.

The Importance of Structure

In the words of one longtime breed-rescue expert, the best thing you can provide for a troubled dog is "structure, structure, structure." Julie Starkweather has been breeding Labrador retrievers since 1970 and placing rescued Labs in new homes since 1987. Many hundreds of dogs have passed through her Connecticut home in that span of time.

"All dogs like structure," she says, "and that is what a pack provides." She explains that abused and/or neglected dogs have normally not had a daily schedule or a place to fit in that is comfortable to them. They do not know what to expect, and their behavior is very much a reflection of this.

Julie has found that abused dogs, even more than neglected dogs, benefit from a daily schedule that is closely adhered to, so that the dog knows from day to day what to expect. This consistency, over time, helps an abused dog gain the security that nothing bad is going to happen to him.

This makes perfect sense. A few hours or days of kindness may be pleasant for an abused dog, but they do not communicate that he is now—and always will be—safe from harm. It is a structured life, with consistency in a daily schedule and in kind handling, that helps a dog understand that his situation is now different. The security that he gains from all of this wonderful predictability is the root of his healing. It will provide the foundation for his ability to be trained and to live peacefully with his adoptive family.

Neglected dogs gain security from a structured life, too. The most difficult dogs in this category are those that were separated too early from mother dog. These dogs often suffer from severe separation anxiety, which, according to Julie, takes the longest to heal. Tips for dealing with separation anxiety are covered in Chapter 13.

Is Healing Possible?

Many times the answer is yes, as long as owners do not expect overnight cures. Healing can take time. Behavioral changes may come slowly, especially if the dog is older.

In preparing this chapter, I had the privilege of going "behind the scenes" to see and hear about abused dogs. One of my visits was to the Humane Society of the Treasure Coast, a well-run and beautiful facility in southern Florida. Abandoned and rescued dogs that arrive here first spend five or more days in a holding area, where their health and behavior are evaluated. No matter what the dog's background, his life there is simple—and structured. For example, a new dog stays in his kennel until he can stop jumping up, out of control. Then he gets time out of the kennel, which includes exercise and play.

If a dog has a shy or fearful reaction to an everyday situation, such as a door slamming or a water bowl dropping, the reaction is essentially ignored. But if the dog ventures out of the corner, attempting to sniff around or meet the staff, the dog is warmly rewarded—with food,

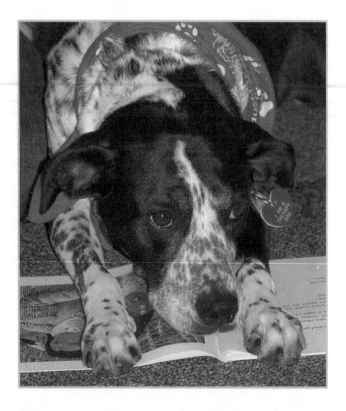

As a young dog, Missy was chronically hit, kicked, and locked in a crate for twenty-two hours a day. Adopted by new owners at age two, she is a testament to the power of careful and loving handling. Missy is now a certified therapy dog, making frequent "friendly visits" to nursing homes, assisted living centers, libraries, and schools. Not only is she healed from her terrible past, she is helping to heal and teach others. She is canine beauty at its finest.

praise, or petting, depending on what the dog can handle. The goal is to help the troubled dog understand that noise and people are "no big deal."

This can take time. The humane society's staff and volunteers will work for days or weeks with a new dog to achieve stability and then to build the dog's confidence. Their goal is to make that dog adoptable, meaning that it can live safely and happily with a new family, even though further training and healing may be needed.

Not all dogs are adoptable, of course. The scars of abuse or neglect may run deep, and the resources of many adoption organizations cannot provide the rehabilitation that some dogs need. Fortunately, most dogs that pass through an adoption organization are screened by experienced people. Those that are likely to fail, because of serious physical or behavioral problems, are not placed. This is not foolproof, of course. Chapter 16 provides help for adoptive owners whose best efforts fail. But you should know that even in the hands of experts, some dogs cannot be saved. Rehabilitation efforts do not always work.

Julie Starkweather points out that a 100 percent change in certain behaviors may not be possible, either. I like her explanation why. "Dogs are like people," she said, "in that they have their own personal likes and dislikes." She gives them the leeway to be individuals.

All dogs, of course, should be taught to meet certain standards of basic good behavior, such as housebreaking skills and responding to a corrective growl—"Nhaa!" But so what if a dog doesn't like to go out in the rain or can't be trusted to stay in the yard without a leash on? One of Julie's male Labs hated puppies to his dying day. Dog personalities are one of the spices of life, in my opinion. It would be a boring world indeed if dogs were all the same.

Medical Intervention

Because dogs do have their own unique personalities, they are affected in different ways by abuse and neglect. Over the years Julie has seen abused dogs that were terribly aggressive and those that were not. She has known dogs that had no abuse in their backgrounds but that had

Should You Adopt an Abused Dog?

Maybe. Not all good dog owners have the ability, interest, and understanding to tackle the job of rehabilitating a troubled animal. The dog's temperament, age, breed (or mix of breeds), health, and rehabilitation requirements also will affect an adoption decision. Consider these points before you decide on adopting an abused dog.

* Have you owned dogs before? A dog with special handling and training needs will probably do best in the hands of an experienced owner. This is not a job for beginners.
* Do you have a lot of available time to spend with a dog? A big part of the healing process is you. Taking care of an abused dog should be a priority, not an afterthought.
* Is your own life structured? A freewheeling, go-with-the-moment lifestyle is not what a troubled dog needs. If structure and routine are not your style, you probably won't find it easy to provide them for a dog, either.
* Are family members agreeable to the adoption? Are they willing to follow your instructions for interacting with the dog?
* Do you have access to support? This might include adoption counselors, breed rescue workers, an experienced trainer, and a trusted veterinarian. You may need to turn to some (or all) of these individuals as you work with your dog.
* Is the dog a good candidate for recovery—or at least significant improvement? I would argue that a middle-aged pit bull used in dogfights has less chance for rehabilitation than a year-old beagle kicked around by an abusive rabbit hunter. Assess the dog's age, breed, and history to get a general idea if the adoption makes sense.
* Are you prepared to euthanize the dog if problems of aggression, emotional instability, or painful illness make this the most humane course of action? Hanging on to a dog with profound, insurmountable problems may indicate that you are unable to be objective about your rehabilitation efforts.

serious, insurmountable aggression problems. Her conclusion after thirty-plus years of working with dogs is that there is a class of dogs that do not see the world the same way as other dogs. If the dog were a person, he or she would probably be classified as paranoid.

Which brings me to an important part of helping a dog with behavioral problems. Brain chemistry, or "wiring" if you will, must be functioning properly for a dog to behave normally—or at least to start learning to behave normally. Without it, an owner's best efforts may fail.

In the last decade, the veterinary community has gathered a great deal of knowledge about canine brain function and how it relates to behavior. Veterinarians have been increasingly successful at using psychoactive drugs to help dogs with serious behavioral problems that do not respond to proper handling, a balanced diet, plenty of exercise, and good training.

I have known or heard about various dogs that suffered panic attacks, chewed open wounds into their paws (self-mutilation), ran constantly in circles, had seizures, chased invisible prey, and dug compulsively on furniture. One mild-mannered dog attempted a sudden lethal attack on its owner. Were these the result of abuse, neglect, or some other stressful situation? Possibly, but it's hard to say. Sometimes genetics and a sensitive personality make a dog susceptible to such problems. In reality, we often can never know why dogs do some of the bizarre things they do. But owners still have a responsibility to respond to the problems.

Fortunately, medical intervention can sometimes help. If your adopted dog is behaving abnormally or is not responding as you might expect to a safe, healthy environment, seek out a veterinarian's advice. You can even ask for a referral to a veterinarian who specializes in behavioral problems. He or she will help you evaluate your dog's behavior and advise whether medication, such as antidepressants, can help.

If you decide to use medication to treat your dog, be prepared to wait weeks or even months for it to work. I am not saying this to be pessimistic. On the contrary, I do support drug intervention for certain behavioral problems. But medication does not offer an overnight cure. You will still need to provide structure, exercise, training, a good diet, supervision, and (this goes without saying) plenty of love and attention.

A Lesson for Life

For several years in the late 1980s and early 1990s, I had the privilege of helping an organization called Adopt-A-Dog, based in Greenwich, Connecticut. This organization is an intermediary between the pet-seeking public and rescue groups, humane societies, and local pounds.

Adopt-A-Dog works like this: Mrs. Smith calls and says that she is looking to adopt a female beagle or beagle mix. She would like a dog between the ages of three and five with a sweet temperament. The Adopt-A-Dog staff use their resources to scour animal rescue organizations in the region to find the appropriate dog for Mrs. Smith. Then they help bring the two together.

Adopt-A-Dog has been successful at finding homes for thousands of dogs. In 2002 it opened its own shelter in nearby New York State.

"Puttin' on the Dog"

Adopt-A-Dog's major annual fund-raiser, called "Puttin' on the Dog," started in 1987. It is a fun, untraditional dog show for pets. For a small entry fee, owners can compete with their dogs in classes like cutest dog, best tail-wagger, best kisser, largest and smallest mutt, etc. Public turnout is great, and the money and publicity generated from the event are used to support some wonderful adoption work.

Here comes the judge

My job each year at "Puttin' on the Dog" was to be one of the judges. The first year I had the dubious honor of deciding which dog was the cutest. You never want to tell two dozen people who are madly in love with their dogs that *theirs* is not the cutest—because really, they are all great. But it was for a good cause, so I agreed to stick my neck out.

After picking an adorable German shorthaired pointer puppy as the winner, I tried to make a quick escape to my car. Before I could get away I was approached by one of the event organizers.

"John, could you please help us? One of our judges didn't show, and we need your help judging another class."

"Of course," I said. "Which one?" I was led to a ring bearing a sign that read "Most Unlikely to Succeed."

"Just ask the owners about their dogs," the woman said, "and give ribbons to the most poignant stories."

I really had no idea what to expect. I walked into the ring to meet nine or ten dogs and their owners. Handlers were chatting happily, and their dogs were calmly sitting by their owners, wagging their tails.

Stories I'll never forget

I asked the first woman about her dog. What was her dog's name? How old was she? Where did she get her? What was Brandy's story?

I learned that Brandy was six years old. She had been rescued two years before in New York City. She had been abused in a cult ritual by human monsters. She was blind, because both of her eyes had been poked out. She was doing well now. She loved her new family, and her new family loved her. She was the best dog in the world, they felt.

This little brown dog licked my face as tears ran down my cheeks. I was overwhelmed. Details of the other horror stories I heard that day are too painful to recount. I was amazed that this group of beautiful, loving dogs had lived through such nightmares. They *all* got ribbons that day.

While I was meeting the dogs, I made it a point to ask each owner what he or she did to help their adopted dog overcome such cruelty. They all said essentially the same thing. "I love him, and I train him, and I provide him with the best life that I can. He is my friend and the most forgiving creature in the world."

It made me think how undeserving we, as a species, are of such forgiveness and devotion from dogs. They never give up on us, which I find overpowering and almost incomprehensible.

Chapter 16

When the Best Efforts Fail

DOG ADOPTION IS an optimistic act. Owners take an unwanted animal into their home and provide it with food, shelter, exercise, training, and love. Most dogs blossom under such circumstances, rewarding their owners with good health, obedience, fun, and companionship.

It is not fun or easy when an owner's best efforts fail. The optimism of adoption coupled with the expenses of food and health care, the hard work of training, and the emotional bonds that develop—these are all difficult to think of as wasted. As a result, owners may prolong a bad or dangerous situation, in the hopes of turning it around. Or they may end the adoption but suffer from profound sadness or guilt over their failure.

A decision to end your dog's adoption—or even to end the dog's life—is almost never an easy one to make. But sometimes it is the right decision. This chapter will give you some guidance if you suspect that your adopted dog will not be able to stay. It will also help you understand your grief after he is gone.

A Good Dog in the Wrong Place

Some people believe that there is no such thing as a dog with a bad temperament. Although I disagree, I do believe that there are dogs with certain personalities that are living in the wrong situations. Does this make for a "bad dog"? Not necessarily.

Take, for example, the field-bred springer spaniel living with the eighty-year-old couple with health problems. This dog is a ball of fire that can run all day. Living with infirm seniors, this springer has a "bad" temperament. But the same dog has a perfect temperament for living with a younger person with a passion for upland bird hunting.

The vicious German shepherd that is perfect at earning his keep behind the fence of a scrap yard would be a disaster living with a family of four in a suburban neighborhood. A noisy, aggressive terrier might be the nightmare resident of a condominium complex. But he could be the star "ratter" living in a big barn or horse stable.

My point is that many problem dogs might be less of a problem—or even an asset—in another setting. Unfortunately, it is not easy to place every mismatched dog into a more appropriate home. But as the owner of a problem dog, you have a responsibility to try.

Fortunately, there are people and organizations that dedicate themselves to helping. They are our humane societies, animal shelters, and breed rescue organizations. Even if your adopted dog did not come from one of these places, they will help you.

But you must help them. Be honest about your dog's strengths and weaknesses. Describe your household and why you think this dog was a poor fit. Never lie about aggression issues, if there are any. The safety of shelter workers and the success of the dog's next adoption may depend on it. Also, maintain your dog's immunizations and provide health records to prove that you have provided good care.

Also, don't wait many months or a year to decide that you have adopted the wrong dog for you. Problems will only get worse over time, not better. Plus, your dog deserves a chance to be in a more appropriate environment, living a happier, more fulfilling life. Have the courage to admit that you cannot meet your dog's needs and act quickly to give him a chance to find someone who can. When you adopt again, use what you have learned to get a better match.

In Sickness and in Health

All dog owners face the possibility that their dog's health will fail. Adoptive owners are no different. If you feel that health issues, including those related to aging, are coming between you and your adopted dog, talk to your veterinarian. He or she can help you better understand your pet's physical state and provide support that may help you deal with the problems.

An infirm dog may simply need medication for arthritis or insulin injections for diabetes. Some behavioral problems are helped by medication. Fleas and mange are treatable; most tumors can be removed. Even amputations, traumatic as they seem, can improve and prolong a dog's life. You can handle these things!

But don't do it alone. Get your veterinarian's help, and talk to adoption workers at your local shelter. They want to see every adoption succeed and will give you valuable advice for managing the care of your sick or aging friend.

Aggression

This is perhaps the biggest problem. Aggressive dogs are dangerous. They should not, in my opinion, be kept as pets in a family home, especially a home with children. Despite valid efforts by adoption workers to screen for aggression problems, some aggressive dogs do end up getting adopted. And when no screening process is in place, such as when you take in a stray or accept a hand-me-down dog, the potential for undetected behavioral problems can be even greater.

Unless a dog is just out-and-out nasty, behavioral problems that include aggression may be difficult to diagnose, especially in a shelter environment. Julie Starkweather, the Labrador retriever breeder and rescuer described in Chapter 15, explains that sometimes the reverse actually happens—a dog may show signs of aggression in a multidog setting (i.e., a shelter, kennel, or pound) but be fine otherwise.

So aggression can be a tricky issue to evaluate accurately. Chapter 10 describes issues of mouthing and biting, which you should read carefully to better assess your dog's behavior. If your dog came from a humane shelter or adoption organization, speak to an adoption counselor about the aggression problems you are seeing. These specialists can also help you determine the seriousness of your problem.

Here are some warning signs that your dog may be aggressive: lip curling, baring the teeth, snapping if awakened suddenly, or growling when made to do something, such as get off the couch, be brushed, have ears cleaned or toenails clipped. Aggression about food is described in detail in Chapter 12.

Why are some dogs like this? We all wish we knew. Abuse and neglect can sometimes cause serious behavioral problems, as described in Chapter 15. I believe dogs can inherit an aggressive temperament, thanks to indiscriminate breeding and aggressive parents. Some breeds were specifically created for work that requires aggressive behaviors. These instincts, gone awry or simply left unchecked by the lack of obedience training, create problem pets. Dog hybrids make the news all too often because of aggression problems. I believe that these part-wolf or part-coyote dogs are not "wired" like a true domestic breed. Their partly wild instincts make them too unpredictable to succeed in a pet home.

And finally there are what I call the "psycho dogs." I've met only a few over the years. These dogs are truly unbalanced and are violently aggressive—some for no apparent reason, others because of neurological problems. The saddest case I remember was a German shepherd puppy. I met this young dog in training class when he was four or five months old. Much of the time he was a sweet, affectionate, and agreeable puppy. Then suddenly he would transform into a snarling, snapping, lunging monster. Healthy, sound puppies don't act like this—ever. I knew something was very wrong, and after a few months of training efforts, so did the owners. No one could ever live safely with this dog. They had him euthanized before he was even a year old.

Euthanasia

Intellectually, we can know that putting a dog to death is more humane than permitting a life of suffering or risking harm to his owners. But anyone who loves dogs feels sadness over the need to inflict death. We are moral people who value life, and euthanasia makes us feel bad. And so it should.

I strongly recommend that you *not* make a euthanasia decision alone. Your adoption counselor, your veterinarian, or an experienced obedience instructor (or all three) can help you evaluate your adopted dog's behaviors and give you a professional opinion about your options. Their expertise and extensive knowledge of dogs will give you a perspective that you probably do not have. If euthanasia seems like the only logical conclusion, then it is probably the right thing to do.

Be reassured that modern euthanasia techniques are quick and painless. I have witnessed it with my own dogs and with dogs in the veterinary hospitals where I have worked. Death comes gently and immediately. The suffering ends. The dangerous aggression ends. Peace comes.

Pet Loss Counseling

Don't let anyone tell you that mourning a pet's death is trivial. It is a profound loss. If you chose euthanasia for your dog, for whatever reason, you are bound to experience some powerful feelings. They may be guilt, regret, sadness, anger, relief, or just about anything else. As an owner of an adopted dog, you may also have feelings of failure or frustration, as you tried to save an animal that turned out not able to be saved. After a dog has been euthanized, it's not uncommon to feel depressed for days or weeks on end. Even other dogs in your household may act depressed. They lost a pack member, too.

You have a right to your feelings, and I encourage you to accept them as a valid part of adjusting to your pet's death. I also encourage you to talk about your feelings to your pet-loving friends and relatives. Avoid those who would trivialize or mock your grief. They will only add embarrassment or shame to your sadness, which is extremely unkind. Mourning the loss of anything beloved is never embarrassing or shameful. To me, it is the sign of a compassionate, sensitive, and loving human being. You are a wonderful person for having cared for and loved your dog.

Don't be afraid to seek help if your grief and mourning get in the way of living. Pet-loss counselors and even regular therapists are trained to help us resolve powerful feelings so that we can get on with the joys of life. Just think: How are you going to give another adopted dog a good home if you cannot see past the previous one's death? Try to put your love of dogs to good use by resolving your grief, gathering your courage, and starting over with a new dog that needs you desperately. There are a lot out there. And one is bound to have you smiling through your tears. That's the power of dogs.

Part Four

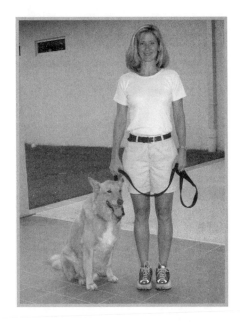

Adoptable Dog Training

With a little basic training, adopted dogs can become great pets. But the training they require often requires extra measures of consistency, patience, and persistence—plus broader thinking in solving problems. These chapters guide you through the basics, with troubleshooting tips in case things go wrong.

Chapter 17

A Commonsense Training Philosophy

MY APPROACH TO obedience training is designed for the average dog owner. It is made up of commonsense training techniques and an easy-to-relate-to philosophical view. My first and foremost goal is to make your job of training your family dog fun and effective.

You do not need complex handling skills or a Ph.D in animal behavior to succeed with these training methods. You simply need to be a person with no more than average skills or intelligence and a modest time commitment to practice the exercises. I have always admitted that I am not highly coordinated, super-smart, or extremely well educated. Yet I have wonderfully trained dogs. You can, too.

In developing this training approach, I have brought together many ideas about how dogs and people learn best. This includes adopted dogs as well. Take a few minutes to read this short chapter. It will give you the mind-set to have great success with your dog.

Motivation to Train

As a longtime dog obedience instructor, I have found that one of the most important things I do is keep my students motivated to train their dogs. After a long day at work or caring for children, most people want to spend their free time reading the newspaper, visiting with friends, or watching television. Practicing Sit-Stay is boring! No one can argue that relaxing with our children and the family dog at the beach is more fun than practicing Come on Command training techniques. Nevertheless, daily practice is imperative if you want to have a well-trained dog.

How do I motivate owners to work with their dogs regularly? By making training fun and by making it as easy as possible to succeed. In other words, I embrace the well-known "K.I.S.S." system. You know: **K**eep **I**t **S**imple, **S**tupid! The less complicated the training procedures, the more willing owners are to practice them. And when training is easy and fun, owners are easily inspired to make dog training a regular part of their lives.

Focused Training

Adoptable Dog training is a pet-oriented program. It is not designed for the obedience trial or agility-ring enthusiast who makes dog training an avocation or a profession. These competitive people learn to master training techniques that require the grace of a ballet dancer with as many arms as an octopus! Leashes, doggie biscuits, clickers, etc. seem to magically materialize in their hands.

I have found that few pet owners are interested in the intricacies of competition training. In fact, about 99 percent of all dog owners are pet owners. They could not care less about the "straight sits" and precision heeling that are required in obedience competition. They just want a dog that is obedient and a joy to live with. And they do not care if their dogs can do agility-ring tricks.

Unfortunately, the vast majority of obedience training classes put an emphasis on competition training. The training tools and techniques in these classes are rooted in competition obedience. It is hard for obedience instructors who are so caught up in their dog hobbies to relate to the needs of pet owners.

The result is that too few dogs and owners are getting the type of training that they need. Sadly, many dogs are placed in shelters because their owners could not embrace a complicated training process.

In contrast, my training program focuses solely on the relevant needs of the dog owner looking for a great pet. This in itself is a great motivator for dog owners.

Step-by-Step Techniques

Each obedience exercise in this *Adoptable Dog* training program is broken down into simple components. When an exercise is broken down in this way, success for the dog is easily achieved. When owners see their dogs succeed, they are motivated to continue training. In a step-by-step progression, owners more successfully reach the end result of each obedience exercise with their dog.

There are bonuses along the way. The dog's behavior steadily improves because of the positive interaction that he is having with the owner. Positive interaction with a pack leader and the opportunity to use his brain in a constructive way quickly transform any dog into a more manageable individual. By the time each obedience exercise is mastered, the owner is seeing a new dog.

Effectiveness

It is not enough for training techniques to be just fun and easy. Training techniques must also be effective. The most important motivator is success. Training techniques must be fundamentally sound and proven to work, or owners are just wasting their valuable time. Dogs are not dolphins or seals. They are canines. My training techniques have evolved from a thorough understanding of dogs and how they behave and learn.

A Fundamental Approach

My background with dogs is not academic. I did not learn how to train dogs by sitting in a classroom studying theories of animal behavior. I developed my techniques, philosophies, and opinions from a lifetime of training, observing, hunting, and living with dogs. You may encounter more scholarly texts about canine behavior, but you won't encounter more readable guides for training your own pet. That is an important strength of this approach.

The education of a qualified dog obedience instructor comes from an accumulation of knowledge. One of the ways that I perfected my approach over the years was by reading other people's experiences and opinions about dogs. While reading virtually everything about dogs that I could get my hands on, I culled the rubbish and incorporated what I believed to be plausible and credible into my own training philosophy.

I know that information and training techniques have to do more than just "sound good." My approach avoids trendy and faddish training philosophies. Methods that simply sound good, but in practice are ineffective, are patently avoided.

Avoiding Abuse

Training methods must never be abusive to a dog. Dogs cannot learn when they are being physically or mentally abused and are emotionally out of control. Hitting, kicking, and choking dogs in the name of training—or for any other reason—is an abomination. Unfortunately, techniques that employ abuse have been going on for decades. This type of training may be less prevalent now than it was in the past, but it does still exist.

On the other hand, some newly popular training approaches shun any kind of discipline, however humane. I have heard trainers insist that telling a dog "No!" will hurt his feelings. I have heard that training collars are torturous and that all corrections are nothing more than punishment. I shun training techniques and philosophies that are designed to appeal to and in fact pander to the narrow-minded assumption that any type of discipline is abusive.

Training Through a Canine Point of View

I call my approach "training through a canine point of view." This means that I teach owners to look at the world through the eyes of their dogs. With a new puppy I take the place of mother dog. With an older, adopted dog I become pack leader in ways that a wolf does, as described in Chapter 7.

I sincerely believe that dogs feel that they are the same type of creature that we are. I don't know if dogs feel that they are human or that we humans are dogs, but I'm convinced that they feel we are all the same. Of course, I know that dogs cannot think or learn on a human level. But humans can learn to think like a dog. I have learned from experience that when owners learn to think like a dog, they can train their dogs much more effectively.

Scientists believe that domestic dogs evolved from wolves about ten thousand years ago. Domestic dogs and wolves still have many similar behaviors, which I have learned about in my research on wolves. I sometimes draw parallels between wolf and dog behavior, although I am not a wolf biologist and have not studied wolves in the wild. But my comparisons of wolf and dog behavior make important points. My goal is to help dog owners understand and train their dogs as canines— not humans in little furry suits.

Does this "training through a canine point of view" approach sound new or trendy to you? Although this may be the first time you have thought of interacting with your dog this way, this approach is actually ten thousand years old. It all started the first time wild canines and human beings teamed up to form a bond, living and working together. It's as old as dogs themselves.

It Is Fun and It Works

This commonsense training approach is for the person whose primary desire is to share his or her home and life in harmony with a canine companion. It was created for people who want a dog that is a valued family member not only in their home, but also in their community. It gives owners the skills to train their dog to be responsive to commands and under control in all circumstances. Although the wolf biologist or the Ph.D. behaviorist might question the ideas I have about canines, what they cannot truthfully do is deny that my training techniques are fun and that they work.

Chapter 18

Using the Right Equipment

WHEN I ATTENDED training classes in 1972 with my first dog, Jason, an Irish setter, the only training equipment I needed was a six-foot leash and a choke collar. That's what every dog used and every handler was told to buy.

Since then, training equipment—like everything else in the dog business—has evolved and expanded. Now there are specific training tools designed for different sizes, ages, body shapes, and personalities of dogs. In general, this customized approach is a good thing, but it leaves a lot of room for confusion about what to buy.

Here are in-depth descriptions of training equipment now in common use. These items are widely available through pet supply shops, doggie boutiques, catalogs, and some groomer and veterinarian offices. It is helpful to have an awareness of all this equipment, because some of it is just right for your dog. But which? These guidelines will help any owner match the right equipment to the right dog.

Descriptions of the effectiveness of this equipment are included as well, because some of these inventions are great, while some are garbage. In addition, some training tools can create safety concerns if not used appropriately. You will find that information here, too.

Leashes

Walk into any well-stocked pet supply store and you will quickly discover that your choice of leashes is almost endless. Entire walls are covered with leashes. You can choose one from two feet up to fifteen feet long, including leashes that stretch or extend in that range. You can buy a leash whose width is a skinny eighth of an inch or a hefty inch or more, plus anything in between.

Leashes can be made of leather, cloth, metal, or nylon. You can have any color that you can think of, plus prints with themes that range from psychedelic to patriotic. Some leashes come with little embroidered whales, paw prints, or palm trees on them. I've even seen diamond-studded leashes. Some have fake stones and—in Nantucket or Palm Beach—real stones!

The six-foot training leash

After a dog is properly trained for the Controlled Walking exercise, the type or length of leash that you use is irrelevant. A trained dog will understand what is expected of him, and he will respond properly no matter what type of leash is attached to his collar. That is the time to

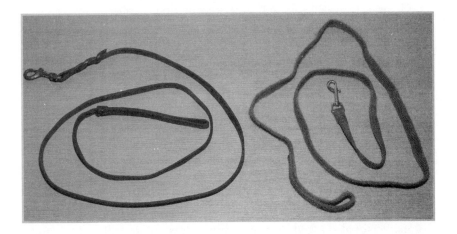

Your training leash should be six feet long and made of cloth, leather, or nylon. Avoid metal leashes and expandable leashes for training purposes.

indulge your fancy for whales or rhinestones if you like the idea of a decorative leash. It's also the time to get a retractable leash (the kind that unwinds and extends out of a plastic casing) if you like a bit of gadgetry.

But for training purposes you need a six-foot, fixed-length leash. Six feet is the length that is best suited for carrying out obedience training techniques. The dog is kept close to you but still has a little room to maneuver. The leash can be gathered easily into one hand or extended out, depending on the exercise. After thirty years of teaching dog obedience classes, I have yet to find anything that works better.

Leash materials

Any nonmetallic material is acceptable. I don't like metal leashes for a number of reasons: They are heavy, noisy, and too difficult to fold up in your hands. The leashes made of twisted wire (usually in a plastic coating) are too stiff. A softer material that is easy to handle works best.

I personally prefer a leather leash. Once broken in, a leather leash feels great in your hands. Maybe my days of playing city-league soft-ball gave me a fondness for this piece of equipment, because nothing feels better than a well-oiled, broken-in baseball glove! When well cared for, a leather leash will outlast your dog. In fact, Barbara saved the two leather leashes from her beloved Labs as mementos of their many years together. But beware, a dog with a chewing habit (or an untrained puppy) is not a good candidate for leather. Your investment will be wasted if the leash is chewed in half.

My second choice is a six-foot cloth or canvas leash. These, too, are comfortable to work with, and they are much less expensive than leather leashes. They can be washed easily if mud, salt water, or sand get on them.

Many people purchase and like nylon training leashes. These are made of that shiny, slippery woven fabric that comes in a rainbow of colors. Personally, I find that most nylon leashes are stiff in my hands. They are uncomfortable, because the edges feel sharp and abrade against my skin. However, I do allow my students to use them if that is their choice. As long as a handler finds a nylon leash comfortable, it will serve the purpose.

Leash width

Two factors will determine the appropriate leash width. The first is what feels comfortable in your hands. The second is the size of the dog that you are training. A person with small hands and a Yorkie is generally better off with a thin leash. An individual with large hands and a bull mastiff would be better served by a wide leash. These are extremes, of course. The choice really boils down to what the handler feels most comfortable using.

A word about retractable leashes

A retractable leash is a twenty-foot leash encased in a plastic holder. A button on the holder is pushed to let the leash out and another to automatically wind the leash in. You can adjust the leash's length to suit your need.

I have often said, "I hate retractable leashes but I wish I had invented them." That's because there are about nine million of them out there. Personally I don't like them for a number of reasons. I find them cumbersome. I accidentally dropped one and the plastic handle smashed.

I also find that many of the people who use these leashes do not have much control over their dogs. These owners allow the dogs to extend the leash way too far at inappropriate times and places. I have had "leashed" dogs come running up to me from twenty feet away on the beach, frightening my young child or tangling up in my dog's six-foot leash. I have seen owners on busy city streets let their dogs pull way ahead, putting other pedestrians at risk.

Nevertheless, many people love retractable leashes. If you do, too, great. However, retractable leashes are not training tools. They are way too awkward to use to teach obedience exercises. Once your dog is trained, you may find the retractable leash handy. Just be sure to use it cautiously.

Regular Collars

There may be even more designer collar choices available for your dog than there are leashes. You can even get leashes and collars that match. But I won't get too descriptive here. I will stay focused on what type of collar is appropriate as a training tool.

Everyday buckle or snap-clip collars

Every dog should have and wear a buckle or snap-clip collar. Attached to the ring should be an identification tag and the rabies tag from your veterinarian. This is not training equipment; it's safety equipment. (Other collars are described later in this section.) It provides a good

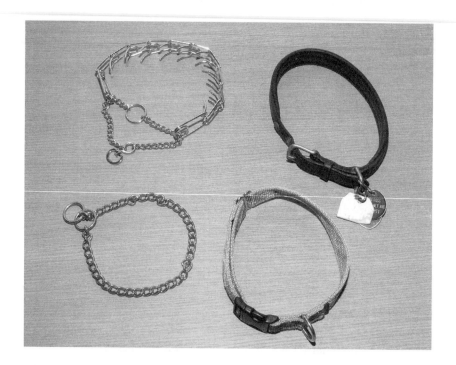

All dogs should wear a buckle or clip collar (on right, top, and bottom), which carries their identification tag. Depending on the dog, this collar can also be used for training, although a training collar (bottom left) or a pinch collar (top left) is usually more effective.

chance that a dog who wanders from its yard, pushes through a screen door during a thunderstorm, or bolts out of the car after a traffic accident will be returned to you. Life is full of such unpredictable events. None of us can assume that a good leash and a fenced yard will *always* keep our dogs under our control. Attach some identification to your pet (cats, too!). You don't want your adopted dog to become homeless again simply because *you* couldn't be found. An ID tag attached to a buckle collar will prevent that.

I have no particular preference when it comes to flat, round, buckle, or snap-clip styles. My springer spaniel, Crea, has several of each. In the summertime in New England she wears a round leather buckle collar. During the school year in southern Florida, she wears a cloth snap-clip collar with a tropical design. She also has a collar with little striped bass on it, an official Jimmy Buffett Parrot Head dog collar, and a bright orange collar for pheasant hunting. A girl must have choices! Now, if I could only have such a nice selection of fly-fishing rods. . . .

Buckle or snap-clip collar for training

Even though the primary purpose of your dog's "everyday collar" is to hold ID and rabies tags, this type of collar may be the appropriate tool to train some dogs. The dog's sensitivity to pain is the determining factor (actually, "discomfort" is a more accurate word—no pain should be involved!).

I had an assistant in Connecticut who very effectively trained her big male collie using a buckle collar. Riley was an extremely pain-sensitive dog and would yip even when gently corrected with a training collar. He was perfectly responsive to gentle corrections on his buckle collar, so that's what my assistant used with this individual. While it is untypical to find a large breed that is this pain-sensitive, it's not unheard-of. Some dogs are better served when trained with a buckle or snap-clip collar.

How will you know? A dog's willingness to respond consistently with a buckle collar will be one indicator. Another will be a frightened or painful response to a standard training collar, such as Riley had. A third factor comes into play with adopted dogs. Most adolescent and adult dogs have had some previous experience with wearing a collar. Perhaps they had a little obedience training. Maybe they wore a buckle collar around the neighborhood. Perhaps a collar only went on their necks for a trip to the vet or the boarding kennel or the local pound. At worst, the dog was beaten with his collar and has a horrible association with it.

One of your jobs as an adopted dog's owner is to stabilize your dog's life and help him to be as well-adjusted and normal as possible. If it takes you a month to get your dog to relax while wearing a soft, comfortable collar, don't despair. *That's training, too.* Focus on one goal at a time, and you will improve your chances for success.

A final thought on these collars. If you have any collar-related information about your adopted dog's previous life, put it to use. If a previous abusive owner had the dog wearing a rolled leather collar, choose a flat nylon one. If the dog spent weeks wandering the streets wearing a piece of clothesline around his neck, don't even consider using an improvised rope collar. You are giving your adopted dog a new life. Use this small but (to me) symbolic item to show that. It may not matter to many dogs, but to certain ones it might be a small sign of hope after months or years of despair.

Training Collars

A training collar is a straight length of chain with a ring on each end. It is the appropriate collar for training most dogs. Cloth versions of training collars are available, but they are ineffective because they don't slide sufficiently for training purposes. I don't recommend them.

If you have never handled a training collar, it probably looks like a puzzle or magic trick. To form the circular collar from this straight chain, hold one ring at about eye level, and allow the chain to hang down. Grasp the bottom ring to steady it, and slowly lower your upper hand, dropping the entire section of chain through the center of the bottom ring. The circular collar is formed, and it simply slides over the dog's head (see photo on next page). The leash attaches to the top ring (the one *without* the chain passing through its center).

Correct link size

Training collars are made of chain links, which come in four sizes. Manufacturers usually label these links as fine, medium, heavy, and extra heavy. I recommend only the two middle sizes (medium and heavy) for any breed of dog. I have found that the fine-linked training collars are somewhat sharp-edged. They can leave sore, red marks on the dog's neck. Extra-heavy links get stuck on themselves, preventing the collar from sliding smoothly and releasing the way it should.

So making your choice of link size is pretty easy. If you have a small or medium-sized dog, use a medium-linked training collar. If you have a large or giant-sized dog, use a heavy-linked training collar.

A properly fitted training collar

The length of this collar must be determined somewhat carefully. If it is too short, the collar won't fit over your dog's head or will be danger-

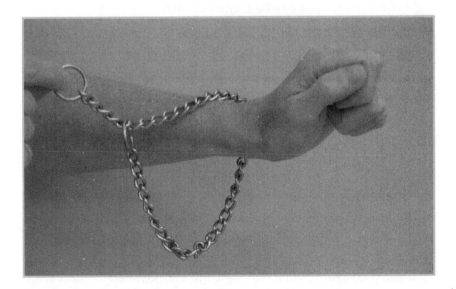

A training collar is properly positioned on a dog when the leash ring (where the leash attaches) is on the dog's right side. The length of chain attached to that ring must first pass across the back of the dog's neck, not under his throat.

ously tight. If it is too long, it won't release properly during the training exercises and will confuse the dog with inappropriate corrections.

For owners of puppies and adolescent dogs: Be prepared to buy more than one training collar over the next year. The collar must fit the dog *now*. Growing into a collar that is too big doesn't work, for the reasons described above. Ask a few dog-owning friends if they have any training collars that were outgrown—you might get lucky and save a few dollars. Otherwise, bite the bullet and buy the right equipment.

The best way to get a proper fit is to take your dog to the pet supply shop. Many now allow dogs inside, which of course makes sense. When the training collar is on your dog, slide your finger through the ring where the leash will attach. Pull up gently. The amount of extra chain extending between your finger and your dog's neck is the determining factor. You should have between two and three inches of excess chain. Remember, if the collar is too long or too short it will not work properly as a training tool.

"I thought it was called a choke collar"

For many years, even the manufacturers who made training collars packaged them as choke collars. I always thought this was misleading and incorrect. This type of collar will choke a dog only when it is used either incorrectly or inappropriately. No humane person buys this collar to choke a dog!

If you allow the dog to pull steadily on the leash while wearing a training collar, the collar *will* tighten around the dog's throat and choke him. (You should teach your dog to walk on a leash without pulling; see Chapter 25.) If you lift the dog off his feet, a training collar will act like a noose and could even strangle him. These are incorrect and inappropriate uses of any collar. Never, ever listen to any training advice that suggests either of these harmful techniques.

When used properly, the training collar has no choking effect at all. It pulls momentarily across the muscular back of the dog's neck in a procedure called a jerk-and-release. Is it bothersome to the dog? Yes. Is it somewhat uncomfortable? Yes. Is it something the dog would like to avoid? Yes. Because of this, the jerk-and-release is one type of correction for an unwanted behavior. As part of a well-designed training program, this correction, when used at the appropriate time and place, helps reinforce learning.

Avoid overcorrections

The back of the neck is one of the dog's toughest body areas. Nevertheless, collar corrections should never be given in a rough or harsh way. Violent jerks and releases on a training collar (or for that matter on a buckle or snap-clip collar) can injure the vertebrae in the dog's neck or back. The dog's front legs should never be pulled up off the ground. *Any* collar correction that causes the dog to yip in pain is an overcorrection. If your dog is yipping in pain, he is being hurt and as a result will not be in emotional control. Dogs cannot learn when they are not in emotional control.

It's all in the teaching

I attended a seminar a couple of years ago given by a trainer who claimed to be nationally recognized. I was curious to hear what he had to say, because I had never heard of him. He said that he did not like training collars because, he claimed, only two out of every fifty of his students could learn how to use them effectively without choking their dogs. I found this fascinating and somewhat ridiculous. In fact, my first thought was, "Boy, this guy is a lousy obedience instructor."

In the way that I teach Controlled Walking and other leash-handling skills, I have found that only one out of every hundred students has trouble learning to use a training collar properly. And I have never had a student choke or injure a dog with a training collar in my classes.

Pinch or Prong Collars

One of the most misunderstood training tools available is the pinch collar, also called a prong collar. The reason for this is the way the collar looks. Quite frankly, it looks like a medieval torture device! The first reaction that most people have is that the pinch collar looks like a spiked collar. It is not a spiked collar, which has points that poke into the dog's neck. The prongs on a pinch collar are not designed to stick into or pierce the dog's skin. They are, quite literally, designed to pinch the surface skin around the dog's neck.

"Ouch! That must hurt"

The pinching correction delivered by a pinch collar is painful to all but the most pain-*in*sensitive dogs. However, to the pain-insensitive dog the correction of this collar is merely bothersome. That's the desired reaction, the reaction that most dogs have to the more widely used training collar.

The pinch collar is an extremely inappropriate training tool for dogs that are even moderately sensitive to pain. Such dogs will yip in pain when given a correction on a pinch collar. If your dog is yipping in pain, he is being hurt, not trained. Keep this collar off any dog that reacts to it in this way.

Who gets a pinch collar?

I never badger or pressure students into doing anything with their dogs that they are uncomfortable with. Most of the dogs that I work with start off with a training collar. I educate my students about pinch collars, and, more often than not, they tell *me* if their dog needs one. The conversation often goes like this:

Student: "I'm having trouble with Controlled Walking with Sparky."

John Ross: "What's going on?"

Student: "He does not feel the correction. No matter how many times I jerk and release the training collar, he ignores me and keeps pulling the leash tight. I'm jerking pretty hard. You told me not to jerk his front feet off the ground. Can we try the pinch collar?"

John Ross: "Absolutely."

When we put a pinch collar on this type of dog, the response is remarkable. The owner suddenly has the ability to give a correction that is bothersome to the dog without hurting him. The dog wants to avoid the correction and therefore stops pulling on the leash. In time, the dog develops a solid habit of Controlled Walking whenever he is on the leash.

A pinch-collar story

I can think of only one time that on the very first obedience lesson I recommended to a dog's owner that a pinch collar would be needed to successfully teach Controlled Walking. The dog was an adopted two-year-old black Labrador retriever–Rhodesian ridgeback mix, named Blacky. He was tall for the breed and weighed ninety pounds. He was solid muscle without an ounce of fat on him. The owner could barely hold him on the leash in class.

I asked the handler to remain after class until everyone else left. I then asked if I could handle the dog. Blacky totally ignored the jerk-and-release corrections when I handled him. I said to his owner, "I recommend that you try a pinch collar." His owner said, "What is a pinch collar?" I pulled one out of my training bag and showed it to the owner. The owner's response was, "I'm not going to stick that thing on my dog." I said, "Fine. I might be wrong. Go home and practice Controlled Walking every day, and maybe he will improve." Quite frankly, I did not believe that he would improve, but you never know until you try.

Things did not improve very much, if at all, over the next two weeks. On the third lesson the owner approached me before the class began. He said, "Listen, I think you were right about the pinch collar. I have been practicing with Blacky every day before and after work, but he is not improving. He does not care about the corrections. Last night when my wife tried to take him out on the leash before bed-time, he spotted my neighbor's dog and dragged my wife across the lawn on her chest. She really wants me to try the pinch collar."

Not a magic solution—but it can be close

I put the pinch collar on Blacky and walked him around the training room. After a few jerks and releases, I could see that I was getting his attention. His owner tried walking him and also felt that Blacky was more responsive.

The pinch collar is not a magic solution or a substitute for training, however. Handlers must still perform the Controlled Walking technique properly and practice with their dogs in order to form a habit. Blacky was much better in class that evening. He paid more attention to his owner and was generally less of a handful. I sent the collar home with Blacky and his owner to try until our next meeting.

The next week Blacky walked into class for the first time without pulling on the leash. I asked the owner, "How is the pinch collar working?"

He replied with the best description I've ever heard of a pinch collar's effectiveness: "Power steering!"

Sure enough, Blacky continued to improve each week. By the end of the eight-week course he walked on the leash as well as any dog in the class.

Why are some dogs insensitive to pain?

A dog's selective breeding has a great influence on its tolerance for discomfort. Labrador retrievers are a good example. In fact, Labs are the breed that most typically requires a pinch collar in my classes. Look at the background of this breed. A hundred years ago, Labs were bred to do one thing: retrieve waterfowl. This required diving into icy water. The dogs that put a paw in the water and said, "No way!" were not the ones that were bred. Only the most stoic dogs were. This produced a breed of physically tough individuals.

A number of other breeds have similar histories, such as other sporting dogs, herding breeds, and hounds. If your dog is one of these breeds or a mix of these breeds, it is possible that a pinch collar will be the appropriate training tool.

The proper pinch collar

Pinch collars are made of small, medium, or large links. I recommend the small links for all dogs. Each link on the pinch collar pops on and off, so that you can adjust the length of the collar to fit any neck. Small-linked pinch collars are the most effective. We feel a small pinch more than a large one. Also, small-linked pinch collars weigh less. The medium- and large-sized collars are heavy, and the dog is extremely aware when it is on. The lighter the collar, the smoother the transition will be from a pinch collar to another type of collar.

Occasionally in the last thirty years I have met dogs of many different breeds that were so wild, large, and strong that they would bend small-link pinch collars with their jumping or lunging. In these situations, despite the drawbacks, I have recommended starting with a medium-link collar. However, as soon as the dogs were responding well and under control, I weaned them onto a small-link collar. In fact, as training progresses, many dogs can even move to the training collar.

The protest yipper

If a dog is yipping in pain he is not the right candidate for a pinch collar. However, some dogs that are appropriate candidates may initially yip in protest.

Here is the typical demographic of protest yippers. They are large, strong, and wild and have a history of dragging their owners around at the end of the leash. These dogs become so exasperated by the fact that suddenly the owner can give a bothersome correction that they yip in frustration. Protest yippers may even resort to jumping on their handlers or nipping at them.

If you are uncertain that the collar is right for your dog or you are getting an adverse response, set up an appointment with a qualified dog obedience instructor.

Correct fit

Pinch collars need to fit properly in order to work effectively. The pinch collar should be loose enough that you can easily slide your hand under it, between the collar and the dog's neck. If it is too tight it will not be able to pinch surface skin around the neck, and it will feel uncomfortable to the dog. If the pinch collar is so loose that it can flip over (so that the prongs are pointing out), it will be completely ineffective.

Are pinch collars safe?

Training collars can constrict around a dog's neck and choke. Dogs have accidentally hung themselves and choked to death on training collars. But pinch collars do not constrict or choke. They simply pinch surface skin. I have never seen a pinch collar leave a cut, abrasion, or a red mark on a dog's neck. Nevertheless, when I am not training my dog I take her pinch collar off. I also recommend removing the pinch collar whenever you crate your dog or leave him home alone. It is possible that if a dog caught the pinch collar on something and struggled, he could hurt himself.

The little black rubber tips

You may have seen pinch collars with black rubber tips covering the prongs. In the late 1980s I was living and training dogs in Connecticut. One day when I walked into a pet supply store to buy dog food, I was approached by the manager, who was a friend of mine. He showed me a pinch collar with little black rubber tips on the prongs. When I asked what it was about he told me that the collar manufacturer was attempting to make the pinch collar appear less fearsome to the general public. The manufacturer felt that the little black rubber tips took away the spiked-collar look. The store manager asked me if I would take one and work some dogs on it and let him know what I thought. I took the collar and tried it on three or four dogs that week and concluded that the little black rubber tips essentially nullified the effectiveness of the pinch collar, rendering it useless.

But in one small way the little black rubber tips are not a complete waste. They can help keep the collar on. Occasionally, small-linked pinch collars can spontaneously pop off a dog. As you repeatedly put on and remove the collar, the link that you squeeze will eventually become loose. When one of the two links right next to the small chain area becomes too loose, the collar can come apart.

Fortunately, there are ways to keep this from happening. First, always take the collar off and put it on using a link somewhere in the middle of the collar. I have never seen the collar come apart on its own from the middle. It is always the loose end links that cause the collar to pop off.

Second, when you get your pinch collar, purchase four little black rubber tips and put them on the two links on either side of the small chain area where you attach the leash. This will prevent these links from sliding apart easily.

Need more help?

You may be able to determine if your dog is the appropriate candidate for a pinch collar by using the guidelines outlined here. However, if you are not sure or there is any question in your mind, find a qualified dog obedience instructor to help you. Be sure that the instructor has experience using the pinch collar. There are people teaching dog obedience classes who have never trained with a pinch collar and have the same misinformed prejudices, based on the collar's appearance, that many pet owners have.

The No-Pull Harness

I like the no-pull harness. For particular types of dogs it is an extremely useful training tool. It has a snap-clip collar, with cords that run from the front of the collar and then under the dog's front legs (his "armpits"). The cords reattach to a ring at the back of the collar between the dog's shoulder blades. The leash attaches to this ring. When you give a jerk and release, the cords give a correction under the dog's front legs.

The no-pull harness corrects in the same manner as a training collar but does not have the potential to choke the dog. Interestingly, even though the no-pull cannot choke the dog, the correction that it delivers is more bothersome to dogs than that of a properly used training collar. This is because the skin under the dog's front legs is more sensitive than the muscular hide at the back of the neck. This makes the no-pull a good choice for what I call borderline dogs. These are dogs that have enough pain tolerance that a training collar is not very effective, yet they may be too sensitive for a pinch collar. The borderline pain-tolerance dog is uncommon, but there are some out there.

Pug faces and the like

I like the no-pull harness for any of the breeds that have pushed-in noses. Breeds such as the bulldog, pug, and Pekinese have enough breathing problems without having a collar inadvertently constricting around their neck. I also think that the no-pull is a good choice when training a dachshund. I worry about the back and neck problems that dachshunds are prone to have. Even when training with a no-pull, you must be sure that your corrections are not harsh and jarring.

Downsides to the no-pull harness

I have found only a couple of faults with the no-pull harness. One has to do with its fundamental design. I find it awkward to perform some of the techniques in my training program. However, with about 85 percent of my techniques it works fine. The other problem is that I find it somewhat complicated to put on. However, keep in mind that I am a mechanical idiot and even have trouble putting a traditional halter on a dog.

Traditional Halters

Traditional halters fit around the dog's shoulder blades and buckle under his torso. They do not work in the same way as a no-pull harness. Traditional harnesses are not designed to give a correction. They are essentially designed for the dog to pull. Handlers use halters on sled dogs to pull the sled. Guide dogs for the blind wear halters to gently pull the handler in safe directions. Whenever you see large pet dogs, such as Labrador or golden retrievers, wearing a harness, you most often see an owner being dragged along behind. The traditional harness is not a good training tool, especially for teaching Controlled Walking.

Head Halters

Head halters fit around the dog's muzzle and clip on at the neck. They work in the same manner that a halter does on a horse. You pull the head in the direction that you want to go. Where the head goes the body follows. A child can guide a horse on a halter, and the same is true for a dog.

Train, don't restrain

I rarely use head halters for one basic reason. I am in the business of training dogs. Head halters are not a training tool. They are a restraint mechanism. To be fair, I have to admit that head halters do stop dogs from pulling. However, they do so by restraining the dog. The problem I have with this is that when you restrain a dog you teach him nothing. I believe that you can successfully walk a dog for six years using a head halter and he will never learn not to pull. The minute you put him on any other type of collar he will pull on the leash.

Another reason why head halters stop dogs from pulling is that dogs become submissive when muzzled. Any experienced veterinarian knows that when you muzzle an unruly, biting dog he will submit and let you handle him. Again, the muzzle will teach the dog nothing. You can muzzle him every time you handle him, but he will still bite you if you try to handle him unmuzzled.

Other disadvantages of head halters

I find head halters abominable to look at. To me, they look like a muzzle. The users of head halters spend a countless amount of time explaining to the public that their dog is not mean and that he is not wearing a muzzle. I would find it tiresome defending a device that is ineffective as a training tool.

Another disadvantage is that almost all dogs initially resist wearing a head halter. While it is true that most dogs adjust, I've had some owners tell me that their dogs never got used to it.

Head halters are not without safety concerns. Because the head halter pulls the dog's head sideways, handlers have to be careful never to jerk on the leash or allow the dog to make a sudden lunge to the end of the leash. Serious neck injury could result.

A place in the universe

Although I am not a fan of head halters, I do recommend them on occasion. One situation comes to mind. I had as clients a lovely couple who owned a golden retriever. They were a frail duo in their mid-eighties. Their dog was a high-spirited ten-month-old. They did not have the physical ability to train this dog to do Controlled Walking. They only needed to walk the dog a few times a day into their yard to urinate and defecate. They had a rather hard time getting the head halter on the dog, and they, too, hated the way it looked. But it did solve their pulling problem.

Nevertheless, when I see an able-bodied person walking a dog using a head halter, I shake my head in dismay. A dog that has learned how to walk on a leash properly is much easier to live with than one that must be restrained every time you step out the front door.

What Does Your Adoptable Dog Need?

Start simple. As soon as possible, get a buckle or snap collar and attach your dog's ID tags to them. Add an appropriate training collar and a six-foot leash as soon as you are ready to start with *Adoptable Dog* training. I hope that is today! The sooner you get training, the sooner your adopted dog will become a well-behaved, great companion.

Chapter 19

Your Training Environment

NOT ALL SETTINGS are created equal—for training a dog, that is. And not all dogs are alike, especially adopted dogs. They come into our lives with a variety of ages, health conditions, personality quirks, and previous training experience. All of these variables require their new owners to figure out what works best for their dog.

For most adopted dogs, training should start at home. That's where you are asking your new family member to live for the rest of his life. Simply getting used to you and your house and the household routines will be part of your dog's initial training. As described in Chapter 8, "Bonding from Day One," your job is to help the dog's transition into your life be as smooth as possible. Your goal is to end up with a dog that is bonded with you and is as comfortable living in your house as you are.

So, your house is where training begins. Behaviors such as housebreaking (if needed), walking calmly on a leash, lying down and staying in place, greeting visitors without jumping all over them, and coming when called all should be taught in your house and yard.

Will your dog be able to behave well everywhere? Yes, eventually. But good behavior at home is crucial. For one thing, it will determine for many owners whether their adoptee is going to stay. So in the grand scheme of things, household manners deserve immediate attention.

Start with this book

The chapters in this section will provide you with all the information you need to teach basic obedience skills to your adopted dog. Depending on your dog's background, you may find that your adoptee knows almost nothing. If that is the case, you will need to work diligently with each of the training exercises found throughout this book.

It is also possible that your adoptee knows too much—of the wrong kinds of behaviors! He may have lots of bad habits. Your job is twofold: Teach good habits and eliminate the bad.

Some dogs come into our lives with a little (and sometimes a lot) of previous obedience training. Lucky you. You just need to fine-tune these basic skills, teaching your new dog that he needs to obey the commands now coming from you.

Keep in mind that canine obedience is based on a relationship with a pack leader. Previous training was not "programming" as one might program a computer. Yes, a trained dog has been taught specific skills. But his willingness to carry them out will depend partly on your ability to take a leadership role and enforce his compliance. It will also depend on his personality, the quality of his previous obedience training, and to some degree on his age and health. So even if you adopt a well-trained dog, be prepared for at least a little obedience work to attune him to you.

Helping Your Dog Learn at Home

The environment that you create in your home will either help or hinder your dog during training. It is an important component in success. It will influence how much *you* enjoy the training process as well.

Here is a description of a bad training environment. The television is on. There is a leftover sandwich on the coffee table. The kids and some neighborhood friends are running around in the next room. You are tired and cranky because it's almost time to start making dinner. It's been raining and the dog has not had a walk or any exercise in two days.

The first three items (television, sandwich, and playful kids) are enormous distractions for most untrained dogs. The noise, food smells, and running around will pull your dog's attention away from the lessons at hand. Owner fatigue and/or a bad attitude are a surefire way to make training feel like torture for you, which the dog will certainly sense. And any dog that needs exercise plus a chance to empty his bladder and bowels is not going to be very calm and attentive during obedience practice.

Let's change this scenario around into a good training environment. The household is quiet. Food and drink are cleaned up. The kids are at school. You planned your day so that the training session fits comfortably into your schedule. You even managed to take the dog for a walk this morning when the rain lightened up.

Great! A short fifteen or twenty minutes are all you need to practice a few steps on several obedience exercises. If you can do this every day—or at least four or five days a week—you are going to quickly and efficiently train your new dog.

Training Classes

Group classes are a place where literally thousands of owners learn how to handle and train their dogs. A great many adopted dogs attend these classes, and they have a great track record for success.

You can find group classes at community centers, in adult education programs, at humane societies, and at some pet supply stores. Veterinary offices and grooming shops also may sponsor classes. And, of course, check your local phone directory.

Group obedience classes help owners in a number of ways. In addition to providing practical instruction, weekly sessions can give structure to an owner's training routine. The take-home assignments become specific tasks to fulfill before the next meeting.

Many of my students tell me that signing up for a class helps them stay motivated to stick with their goal of training their dog. I will be the first to admit that it can be easy to let our busy lives squeeze out any spare time for practicing obedience exercises. Many people have difficulty simply walking their dog each day! I do understand that training a dog completely on your own can be a challenge. So when you and your dog are on an instructor's attendance list—and you spent money to be there—the motivation to attend and participate can be strong. A group class can be the difference between a halfhearted attempt at training and unqualified success.

Many dog owners also enjoy the camaraderie of a group obedience class. There's nothing like a half-dozen other untrained dogs (and their frustrated owners) to make you feel less exasperated about your own mutt. Students from some of my group classes have met outside of class to exercise their dogs and practice training together. Some have become long-term friends, thanks to their common bond to their dogs.

I like group classes, but they are not for everyone. Would you and your adopted dog benefit from joining a group training class? The answer may be yes, but you must evaluate several important things before making such a decision. The wrong dog in the wrong group class will be more than a waste of your time and money. At best, it will sour you and your dog on obedience training. At worst, it could trigger fearful or aggressive behaviors in a vulnerable dog that is not ready for a group setting.

So first and foremost, evaluate your dog. Ask yourself whether he has achieved (or is in the process of achieving) some very basic skills, such as housebreaking and respecting your corrective growl ("Nhaa!"). A good trainer can help you improve on those skills, of course, but you will enjoy class more if you are not busy mopping up urine or struggling with a wild animal on the end of the leash.

Is your dog dangerously aggressive toward strangers and/or other dogs? A good instructor would never put other students and dogs at risk by allowing a dangerous animal into a group setting. If you suspect your adoptee might potentially be a threat, speak to the instructor and arrange for him or her to evaluate the dog privately. I have met dogs whose inexperienced owners suspected they were too aggressive for my class only to discover that the dog was just big, goofy, and completely untrained. And I have met dogs that were described to me on the phone as "usually not a problem" but had to be permanently removed from my group class at the first meeting because of serious aggression problems.

Is your adopted dog nervous and/or fearful? Group classes can be rowdy if the dogs in it are barkers, if they are strongly playful, if they tend to jump or pull on the leash, etc. A good instructor will maintain order, but each group of dogs and handlers does tend to have its own unique "class personality." I've had a few wild groups over the years and also one memorable class where every dog was a nonbarking, nonjumping example of canine calmness. Most shy dogs can manage just fine in a well-run group class, especially if the class size is kept small (ten dogs or less). It's the dog that panics around strangers or other dogs that is not a good candidate for this training format.

Health issues: Do not bring a sick dog to a group obedience class. Do not bring a dog with fleas or other parasites to a group class. Do not bring an unvaccinated dog into a group setting. And do not bring a female dog that is in estrus ("in heat") to a group class. If your dog is recovering from surgery or an injury, ask your veterinarian when it is safe to join a class. An obedience trainer is not a medical expert. When in doubt about any health issue, ask your veterinarian.

Private Instruction

If your budget allows, private obedience lessons can be a great way to get started with your adopted dog. A good instructor can evaluate your dog's personality, his potential and limitations, his existing obedience skills, and his undesirable behaviors in your house and yard. Then an obedience program can be introduced to help you make quick progress toward your goal of a well-trained dog.

Private instruction focuses solely on your family and your dog. The trainer's time is spent solving your problems, answering your questions, and assisting your family members with training. The trainer's visits are arranged around your schedule and can be modified because of illness, travel, etc. Clearly, private lessons are the customized approach, which many owners like.

Downsides? The cost is prohibitive for many people. Plus there's no chance to meet other dog owners and to build a dog's social skills. Some households are too chaotic for a successful private obedience lesson.

The Qualified Instructor

No training environment will work well if the obedience instructor is a poor one. I wish I could say that this is a profession filled with competent, highly skilled people. It's not. I continue to be amazed at the number of poorly qualified people who sell their services as dog experts.

Fortunately, there *are* qualified people out there. They are dedicated to this profession, and they are doing a great job. I have always encouraged dog owners to look beyond the most convenient and cheapest dog trainer to find the one who is the best around. It is not always easy. And as I have said, a good training book is better than a bad trainer. So skip the class—group or private—if you cannot find an instructor who will be great.

Here are my long-standing guidelines for finding a qualified obedience instructor.

Experience

Dog obedience instructors cannot teach what they do not know. First and foremost, a good instructor must be a good dog trainer. He or she should own a dog (a well-behaved one) and should have plenty of experience training many different dogs. A well-meaning dog owner who merely trained a few of his or her own pets is not a qualified obedience instructor!

Dog training experience can come from a variety of settings. Some trainers work for guide dog schools, police forces, or military organizations. Some trainers gain experience by competing in AKC obedience trials, schutzhund trials, tracking tests, agility competitions, or field trials. While these are not pet-focused environments, they are good settings for learning how to train and handle dogs.

Additional dog-handling skills can be developed by assisting in a veterinary hospital or dog grooming salon, by working on the staff of a boarding kennel, or by volunteering in an animal shelter. Each of these experiences provides the opportunity to interact with hundreds of dogs, giving the trainer a solid understanding of canine behavior and temperament.

Teaching skills

A great dog trainer is not necessarily a great teacher. But that is what an obedience instructor essentially is. Your trainer must teach *you* how to handle and train your own dog. He or she must be articulate, organized, and pleasant to be around. Your questions must be answered thoughtfully, your problems must be given realistic solutions, and your dog must be handled humanely. If the trainer comes to your home, you must feel comfortable and secure with a virtual stranger in your house.

Good obedience instructors work hard at being good teachers. They can adapt their instruction to meet the needs of their students. They continue to perfect their training program to make it as efficient as possible. They encourage their students to succeed and try to make training fun. And they run an organized class, preventing unruly dogs or owners from disrupting others.

I have met far too many poor instructors over the years. Don't let a string of dog training credentials fool you. If the trainer can't teach very well, very little of his or her experience will be passed on to you.

Established reputation

The training and teaching skills described above are not developed overnight. But that does not mean a novice instructor won't be great—or that a long-time veteran of the dog business will be brilliant. Ask to observe a group class. Is the trainer friendly but in charge? Is he or she articulate? Are the training techniques humane and easy to understand? Do the owners and dogs both seem to be enjoying the class? Is the class environment mostly calm and organized?

Answers to these questions will give you a good indication if the course is a quality program and if the instructor is well qualified to teach it. Walk out the door if you feel it is inferior. Don't waste your time or money on a bad or even mediocre class. Training your adopted dog is too important! This may be your dog's last chance for success with a family. Do everything you can to make training a great success.

Chapter 20

Sit on Command

ALMOST EVERY FAMILY DOG in the world has been trained to sit on command. Of course, some dogs respond to the command more promptly and reliably than others. Many dogs require multiple commands before they will comply. But they all can do it. In fact, despite all of the complaints that owners may have about their dogs, they almost always tell me, "He knows Sit."

How is this possible? A good number of puppies spontaneously put their butts on the ground when they hear their name and the command "Sit." If you simply get a puppy's attention, chances are good that he will sit and look up at you. Owners often hold a dog biscuit or squeaky toy while they say "Sit" three or four times. When the object that the owner is holding attracts the puppy's attention, sure enough, he will sit. The owner then praises the pup and gives him the treat to eat or the toy to play with. Before long, the dog will develop a reliable reaction, called a conditioned response, when he hears the command "Sit."

Unfortunately in this scenario, the puppy's conditioned response is not to *immediately* sit on command. The first thing a puppy does when he hears the command is look to see if the owner is holding a biscuit or toy. If the prize is in sight, the dog will sit. If the prize is not in sight, the puppy will usually ignore the command.

My objective is to get the dog to respond immediately to the first and only command. He can expect a reward *after* he has sat. It is defi-

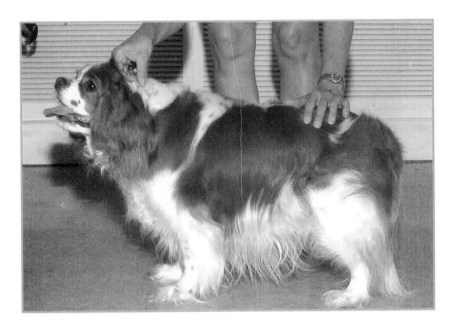

Start teaching Sit on Command by holding your dog's collar in one hand and putting your other hand on his backside.

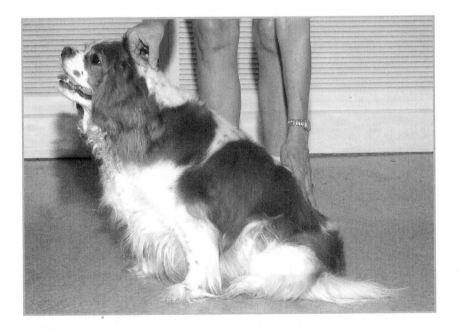

Say "Sit" as you gently pull up on the collar and press him into a sit.

nitely not a situation where the dog is thinking, "Show me the cookie and then I'll do what you want."

While it is true that it is easier to achieve this goal by starting off with a puppy and using proper training techniques from the start, it is never too late. Even if your adopted dog will only sit for a biscuit or requires multiple commands in order to respond, you can still use this chapter to achieve the goal of getting him to sit immediately on the first command.

Is it cruel to compel a dog?

A brief word is needed here about training terminology: Do not be intimidated by it! "Compelling" a dog to do a behavior means to physically force him to do the behavior. Compelling is not rough. Dogs can be compelled in a gentle manner. None of my training methods ever require violent force.

You may hear criticism of compulsive methods. Dog trainers who wish that they could be dolphin trainers seem to take offense to *any* training methods that require compulsion. They want to categorize all compulsive, or force, methods as rough and abusive handling. This is purely propaganda designed to make their training approach seem to be the only reasonable way to train. No skilled dog trainer who has taken the time to hone his or her craft ever brutalizes a dog in training.

Step One: Compelling Your Dog to Sit

* Place your right hand, palm up, through your dog's collar. Your fingers should be pointing toward your dog's tail.
* Place your left hand at the back of your dog's neck.
* Say your dog's name and the command "Sit." After you give the command, pull up and back with your right hand on your dog's collar. Simultaneously slide your left hand down your dog's back along his spine and over his tail, tucking him into a sit. (It does not matter if you choose to place your left hand through the collar and slide your right hand down your dog's back. As long as your arms are not crossed.)

* As soon as he sits, praise him enthusiastically. Be sure to give one command only.

Unlike an eight-week-old puppy that is hearing commands for the first time—and just learning to form associations between signals and behaviors—your adopted dog has heard the command "Sit" many times. Your training goal is not so much to teach him to place his backside on the ground when he hears "Sit" as it is to get him to respond immediately to the first command.

Practicing this compulsive Sit on Command training technique several times a day will help you achieve that goal. Be sure to always give only *one* command whenever you tell your dog to sit. Make sure that every time you give the command you are in a position, with your hands on your dog, to make him comply immediately.

Practice many sits throughout the day. Be sure not to test your dog at this stage of training by giving the command and waiting to see if he will respond. Your job is to help your dog learn to sit immediately when he hears the command. At this time your dog's job is simply to comply, by allowing you to sit him. The only thing your dog can do wrong is to fight, bite, and resist. (See "Troubleshooting" on p. 205.)

Step Two: Inducing Your Dog to Sit

This method uses inducement rather than compulsion. You will be luring your dog to sit instead of compelling him to do so. This method adds animation to the dog's response. It also seems to speed up the learning process.

For this technique you will need an "object of attraction." An object of attraction is simply something that your dog likes and that will hold his attention. It can be a tennis ball, a squeaky toy, or a dog biscuit. Food seems to work the best. Do not use the family cat! Select an object that you can easily hold in one hand and that you can slide into a pocket when not in use.

* Put the leash on your dog and hold it in your left hand. Gather the leash up so that it is rather short. This will prevent your dog from

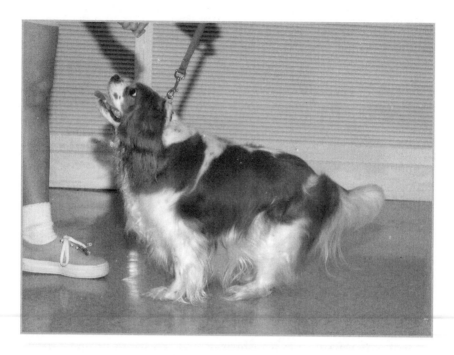

An object of attraction lures a dog into position. Be sure to say "Sit" as you practice this step.

jumping up at the object of attraction if he is an excitable type.

✳ Attract your dog's attention to the object by waving it in front of his nose until he becomes interested in it.

✳ When you have your dog's attention on the object, say "Sit." Then move the object above and behind his head. Holding the object in the correct strategic position behind your dog's head will cause your dog to sit. Be sure to give only *one* command.

✳ If your dog does not follow the object into a sitting position, do not repeat the command. Do not stand there waving the object in his face saying, "Sit. Sit. Sit." Instead, quickly bend over and compel him to sit using the compulsive training technique.

✳ If your dog does follow the object into a sitting position after you say "Sit," praise him enthusiastically.

If this exercise works with your dog it will enhance the training. If your dog does not respond to the inducement method (because he is not interested in any object of attraction), then you can rely exclusively on the compulsive training technique.

If your dog does respond to the inducement method, alternate between inducing and compelling your dog into the sit position. The goal of both of these exercises is to show your dog what you expect him to do when he hears the command "Sit."

If you use a dog biscuit as an object of attraction, it is okay to let your dog eat the treat after every fourth successful repetition. Be sure that you only allow your dog to eat a small amount. You can use a large dog biscuit to attract his attention, but then break off only a small corner to let him eat. If you give your dog a large biscuit after every repetition, you are going to end up with a chubby dog. Too much food reward will also take away your dog's interest in the object of attraction.

If you are using a tennis ball or squeaky toy as an object of attraction, use the same formula. After every fourth successful repetition, let your dog play with the toy for a minute or two. Regardless of what type of object of attraction you choose, pet and verbally praise your dog after every successful repetition.

Step Three: Testing Your Dog

Test your dog with this command by saying his name followed by the command "Sit." If he does not respond immediately, bend over and compel him to sit. Your goal is to condition your dog to respond immediately to the first command. To achieve this you must be consistent with your expectations every time you give a command.

Some dogs will become dependent on having you compel them to sit after the command. If you feel that this is happening with your dog, you will need to use a testing technique that involves a correction when your dog does not respond immediately. The correction should never be given in a harsh way. Corrections do not need to be painful to the dog to be effective. As a matter of fact, overcorrections (those that cause the dog pain) are not only cruel, they are counterproductive to successful training. When dogs are hurting, they are not under emotional control. And when dogs are not under emotional control, their ability to learn is inhibited.

Testing with Corrections

* Start with your dog standing at your left side.
* Gather your leash, so that it is rather short but not tight in your right hand.
* Without touching your dog, place your open left hand, palm down, over your dog's hind end at the base of his tail.
* Call your dog's name and give the command "Sit." If he sits quickly on his own, praise him.
* If he does not respond within a few seconds, give a series of gentle jerks and releases on the collar back toward the dog's tail.
* Do not repeat the command "Sit." Never give more than one command. In order to cause the dog to sit, the jerks that follow should not be straight up but back toward his tail. Be sure not to be rough. Jerk and release just enough to get your dog to sit, but be careful not to jerk too hard. Hard jerks will confuse your dog! If gentle jerks and releases do not cause your dog to sit, this means that he is not ready to test.
* When your dog sits, immediately stop jerking and praise him lavishly.

Practice several sits throughout the day with your dog. Be consistent. Do not test your dog by giving the command without being prepared to give a correction unless you are 100 percent sure he will respond to the first command.

Does the correction bother him?

Several years ago when I was demonstrating the corrective test training technique with my dog for a group class on Nantucket Island, a woman asked a question about the correction. With a somewhat unsure look on her face she asked, "Does that bother him?"

I answered, "Yes. That is what the correction is designed to do, be bothersome to the dog. Never painful. Never hurtful. Just bothersome."

Dogs avoid disagreeable experiences. Certainly they will learn to avoid painful and cruel experiences, too. But along with these extreme

experiences will come backlash effects that are unproductive to training, such as fearing or not trusting the handler. An important part of
good handling skills is learning how to correct a dog effectively without overcorrecting.

Acquiring this skill takes some practice. If it were easy to train dogs,
everyone would have a well-trained dog! And if this were the case, you
probably wouldn't have your adopted dog. Dogs would not be ending
up in shelters as often.

As you practice giving appropriate corrections, do not overcorrect
your dog. Start off easy. If your correction is ineffective, jerk a little
harder. There is no set formula. All dogs are different, but it will not
take you very long to learn what is just right for your dog.

Be sure to release the collar's pressure as soon as you give a jerk-and-
release correction. You never want to gag or choke your dog. And it
goes without saying that you should never hit or kick your dog as a
correction. That's not training; it's abuse.

Trainer's cop-out

Some dog trainers avoid training that involves any corrections, because
it requires practice to carry out techniques with skill. I have read or
heard trainers say, "Oh, it's too complicated for owners to do," or
"Owners will abuse and ruin their dogs trying to master these techniques." Trainers who believe this are just incompetent dog obedience
instructors! After thirty years in this business, I have observed that there
are many good dog trainers who could not teach a *person* anything. And
there are many dog obedience instructors who are ineffective dog trainers. Skills with both dogs and people are necessary to be an effective dog
obedience instructor.

Troubleshooting

What can go wrong with Sit on Command? Probably the most serious problem would be a dog that does not let you handle him. Step
One, compelling your dog, requires you to grasp the dog's collar and
gently pull up while you push down on his backside. If your adopted

dog has never been handled before—or made to do *anything*—this step might cause resistance.

My recommendation would be to ease into handling and also to work on bonding. Stroke your dog, brush or comb him, put his collar on and off a few times, let him eat some kibble from your hand, etc. Take walks together and spend time together in the house. Help him to learn that you will touch him kindly and treat him well.

If these simple activities are impossible to do without the dog growling, snapping, or biting, study Chapter 10 on mouthing and biting and Chapter 16 on adoption failures. Why? Because an obedient dog that is pleasant (and safe) to live with is a dog that accepts handling. A dog that aggressively bites when physically and kindly handled is a serious problem—and a serious liability. Think long and hard about keeping such a pet in your home.

That said, most owners will probably just be dealing with squirming and mild resistance to this exercise. Persevere! Growl "Nhaa!" if necessary. Also, be as smooth and methodical in your handling as you possibly can. Be consistent with your commands. Keep a calm demeanor, even if you are getting exasperated. These qualities will communicate authority to your dog and will help to inspire his respect.

If you find yourself losing patience, end the training session on a successful note. That is, with you in charge. Do not let the dog think that rambunctiousness is the way out of training! Gather your composure, hold the dog's collar, and put him into even a momentary sit. End of exercise. Practice again later in the day, perhaps after the dog gets some exercise and you get some rest.

Be sure your training environment is conducive to success. Distractions such as noise, kids running or playing, food on the table, and other pets nearby can make your dog uninterested or unable to cooperate. Also, be sure the dog has had a bathroom break and some exercise. Small distractions can undo a training session, so try to figure out what they are and eliminate them. It's up to you to help your dog succeed.

Chapter 21

Down on Command

DOWN ON COMMAND means that a dog will lower his body into a lying-down position in response to a specific cue. This cue can be either a verbal command or a hand signal.

Practical Uses

On a few occasions over the years I have had dog owners ask me, "Why does my dog need to learn to lie down on command?" There are both practical and psychological reasons for this important exercise.

In practical terms it is very useful to have a dog that is trained to lie down on command. Whenever I am eating, my springer spaniel, Crea, is attracted to me like a magnet. I tell her, "Crea, go lie down!" She dejectedly flops on the floor nearby and stares at me, her eyes looking up, until every last bite of my food is gone. Her ability to lie down on command makes it easy for me to control her begging behavior.

The skill of lying down on command can come in handy when you wean your adolescent puppy or rehabilitated adopted dog from the kennel crate at night. Many dogs go from being crated in the bedroom to a dog nest on the bedroom floor. At some point during this transition, you will probably find your dog either standing at your bedside staring at you or trying to find a comfortable spot on the bed. A firm "Get on your nest and lie *down*" is extremely useful.

A third example of the usefulness of Down on Command is dog control during a car ride. When your pooch is in the backseat or tail-gate area of your automobile, you cannot drive and physically control him at the same time. "Rover, lie *down!*" can effectively put to an end any unruly behavior that may be brewing behind you.

I can think of many more examples of the usefulness of Down on Command. Your lifestyle and routines will somewhat influence how it is put to use. Also, Down on Command is connected to the obedience exercise called Down-Stay, which is probably the most important skill a companion dog can learn.

That old pack-leader image

Response to the command "Down" is useful not only in practical situations. It is also an indication that the dog views his handler as pack leader. When a dog lowers his body to the ground in response to a verbal command, it is comparable to a submissive dog rolling belly-up to a more dominant dog's growl. It is an indication that your dog acknowledges your authority as his pack leader.

Although Down on Command is not the most difficult obedience exercise for a dog to learn, it can be challenging. That's because it is the exercise that a dominant dog will most likely resist doing. If a dog has the slightest doubt that the handler is the dominant pack member, he will not go down reliably.

Luring a dog down is not the same as getting the dog to respond to a verbal command. A dog may willingly lower his body to the ground when lured by a piece of food or another object of attraction. But do not confuse this response with Down on Command. I've met many dogs that have been trained to follow a biscuit or their owner's hand to the ground. Regardless of how many times this procedure is repeated, this dog will never go down solely on command unless taught to do so.

In many situations, following a hand or biscuit to the ground may serve the purpose. But there will come a time when it is not good enough. Imagine, for example, coming into the house with a bag of groceries in each arm. If you want your dog to lie down, all that would be needed with the well-trained dog is a command, "Rover, down," and the dog is lying down. The cookie-dependent dog cannot be controlled in this situation.

Teach, then test

I take the same approach in training a dog to lie down on command as I do with Sit on Command. First we teach the dog what to do, then we test him.

Step One: Compelling Your Dog to Lie Down

* Begin with your dog sitting at your left side.
* Hook the thumb of your left hand through the top of your dog's collar. The palm of your hand should be open on your dog's back with your fingers pointing toward his tail.
* Slide your right arm under your dog's right leg. With your right hand palm up, grab your dog's left leg. His right leg should be resting on your arm. Lift your dog's left leg off the ground until both legs are in the air.
* Pull back with your left hand on the collar, toward your dog's tail, with enough pressure to keep him in a sitting position. This will prevent him from standing up when you lift his legs.
* Say his name and then the command "Down." After you say the command, gently lower your dog's body to the ground.
* Keep your dog in the down position for a few seconds. Praise your dog enthusiastically and then let him up.

Practice several downs using this technique throughout the day. When you lower your dog's body to the ground, it does not matter if he lies down on his chest, flops on his side, or rolls belly-up. You are just trying to help him understand that the command "Down" means "Lower your body to the ground."

Do not test your dog at this stage of training by giving the command and expecting him to respond properly. Make sure that every time you give the Down command, your hands are on the dog and that you are in a position to make him comply immediately. Show him what you want him to do each and every time he hears the command "Down."

The technique used for Step One of Sit on Command and Down on Command is a compulsive method of training. You are physically compelling your dog to do the behavior after you give the command. In addition to learning how to respond to the command, you are asserting your authority as pack leader, by handling your dog in a gentle but assertive manner. This helps your dog understand that he must take direction from you.

Step Two: Inducing Your Dog to Lie Down

When used properly in a well-rounded training program, inducement training techniques enhance the training process. We will use inducement training to teach your dog Down on Command in the same way that it was used with Sit on Command.

* Start with your dog sitting at your left side.
* Hook the thumb of your left hand through the top of your dog's training collar, the same way that you did when using the compulsive training technique. Place your open palm on your dog's back with your fingers pointing toward his tail. Pull back on the collar to prevent your dog from standing up.
* Get your dog's attention with the object of attraction, held in your right hand. The object can be a dog biscuit, a tennis ball, a squeaky toy, etc. Once you have his attention on the object, say his name followed by the command "Down." Then lower the object straight down from his nose to his toes.
* After your dog follows the object with his nose to the ground, extend the object along the ground in front of him so that he must reach for it.
* When your dog is in the down position, praise him and let him have the object.

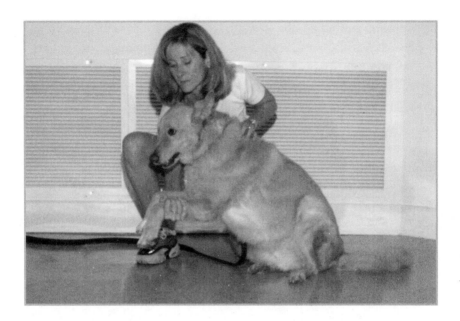

Begin teaching Down on Command by lifting your dog's front legs and lowering him to the ground. Say "Down" as you do so. Be sure to put your other hand on his back to prevent him from standing up.

Give one command only. If your dog does not go down by following the object of attraction, immediately use the Step One training technique and compel him to go down.

Alternate between the Step One compulsive training technique and the Step Two inducement training technique. Do not test your dog at this stage of training by merely using the command "Down" without showing him what you want him to do. Doing so will only slow down the training process. Remember that our goal is a dog that reliably responds to the first command.

Inducement training does not work with all dogs

Dogs that are not food- or toy-oriented do not respond to luring methods. Thank goodness that dogs of this nature are rare. Most dogs live to eat and play! If you own one of these anomalies, you may have to rely solely on compulsive training techniques. However, do not give up easily on trying to find an object of attraction that turns your dog on.

Several years ago I gave private lessons to a woman with a grey-hound. Her dog snubbed every piece of food and every toy we tried. I told her to practice Sit and Down on Command by using the compulsive techniques. I also suggested that she try different things in the hope that the dog would become interested in something.

A few days later the phone rang. Without identifying herself, a woman said, "Hot dogs. He does it for hot dogs." I immediately knew who it was! Since then I have discovered that hot dogs rarely fail. So chop up a nice hot dog (leave off the spicy mustard and chili) for your fussy pup and give it a try.

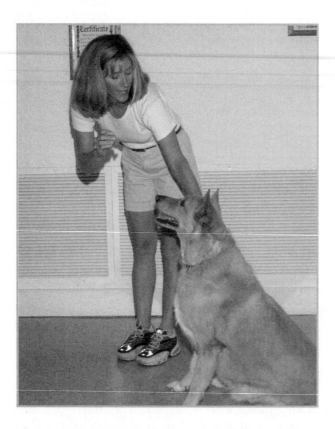

Lure your dog down by using an object of attraction. First get his attention with it, then move it downward below his nose. Bring the treat all the way to the floor so that he lies down to follow it. Be sure to say "Down" each time you practice.

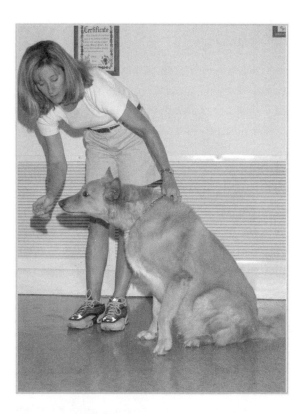

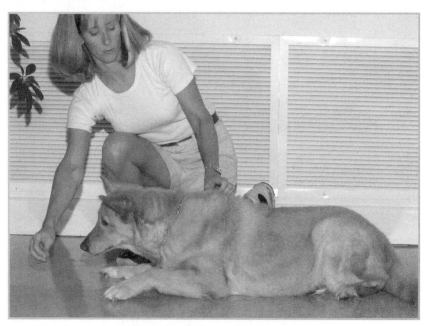

Step Three: Testing Your Dog

After you have spent several weeks with Steps One and Two, teaching your dog what the command "Down" means, you should be ready to test your dog. At the testing stage of training, you can give your dog a correction if he does not respond in the way that you have been showing him all these weeks.

I have to repeat that corrections should *never* be given in a harsh or rough manner. Overcorrections are cruel and unnecessary, and they are also counterproductive. Overcorrections will undermine your training efforts.

Always start off with extremely gentle jerks and releases. If your dog does not respond, jerk and release a little harder. From the time you begin jerking and releasing, it should take no more than ten seconds for your dog to respond by lying down. Ten seconds is a long time!

If he does not go down immediately, do not start jerking harder or begin pushing him down. Do not repeat the "Down" command. Continue to gently jerk and release. If you encounter resistance and he does not lie down within ten seconds, this is an indicator that you need to practice the first two teaching steps for a longer period of time. Continue to show your dog what "Down" means using the Step One and Step Two training techniques for a couple more weeks before testing him again. With practice and patience he will get it.

Testing Technique

* Start with your dog sitting at your left side.
* Gather your leash into your right hand so that you have leverage, but do not make your leash tight.
* Place your left hand, palm down, on your dog's shoulders to prevent him from standing up.
* Call your dog's name and give the command "Down." If the dog does not go down by the time you silently count to three, give a series of gentle jerks and releases toward the ground. Be sure to jerk down and in the direction that your dog's body is leaning.

✳ Give one command only, regardless of how many jerks and releases are needed to get your dog to go down.

✳ Make sure you give an effective correction, but do not overcorrect your dog. Jerk and release just hard enough to get him to go down. If you jerk too hard, you will condition your dog to brace himself for a hard jerk. This would be counterproductive. Gentle jerks and releases will get the job done effectively.

✳ Never pull steadily on the leash. Be sure that you release the collar after every jerk. Pulling on the leash and collar will cause your dog to resist.

✳ When your dog goes down, stop jerking and praise him lavishly. Do not allow momentum to cause you to continue to jerk after your dog is down. Doing so will confuse your dog.

Practice several downs using this technique throughout the day with your dog. Do not test your dog by giving the command without being in a position to give a correction if he does not respond. When you are not doing the Step Three procedure, continue to compel or lure him down using the Step One or Step Two procedures.

Step Four: Testing from in Front

Continue practicing Step Three with your dog at your left side. When your dog has learned to stay in a sitting position (called Sit-Stay and explained in Chapter 22), try this procedure from a new position.

✳ Start with your dog sitting at your left side.

✳ Using both the verbal command and the hand signal, tell your dog, "Stay." Pivot out in front of your dog, leaving a few inches between his nose and your knees.

✳ Gather the leash into your right hand. The leash should be loose, but be sure that you have enough leverage to be able to jerk and release, if necessary.

✳ Place your left hand, palm down, on your dog's shoulders to prevent him from standing up.

* Say your dog's name and give your dog the command "Down." After giving the command, silently count slowly to three. If your dog does not go down by the time you have counted to three, give a series of gentle jerks and releases toward the ground. Continue to jerk and release until your dog goes down.

* Give only one Down command. Do not repeat the command regardless of how many jerks and releases it takes to get your dog down. As soon as your dog is down, stop jerking and praise him lavishly.

Alternate between practicing the testing step of Down on Command with your dog from your left side and from the knees-to-nose position. The objective of this exercise is to condition your dog to drop at the command "Down" in order to avoid the correction and to earn praise.

It is important to keep your left hand on your dog's shoulders when using the Step Three and Four testing techniques. Keep your hand there each time until he is going down on command without having to be corrected. If you do not keep your hand on his shoulders, your dog will probably stand up when you give the collar corrections. Remember to give gentle jerks and releases if you have to correct your dog.

Troubleshooting

Of all the obedience exercises, Down on Command is most likely to bring out some degree of resistance in your dog. This is because a dog must view the handler as pack leader before he will willingly lower himself into this subordinate position.

Mild resistance, such as stiffening the front legs, is just an indication that lots of practice is needed. If the dog is generally willing to be handled and only reluctantly accepts going down, that's no big deal. Spend as many weeks as you need to on the teaching steps and then be methodical on the testing steps. Some dogs will do their best to make you think that doing this exercise is torture. Remind your dog that you are not beating him up! You are just telling him to lie down.

Moderate resistance can come in the form of vocal grumbling.

Grumbling is not something that every dog does, but if you have heard it, you know what I mean. It is not a lip-snarling growl at all. It sounds like complaining. My black Lab, Byron, complained about Down on Command for months. Even into old age, he would occasionally do it. Drifter, my Australian shepherd, had this walrus-sounding grunt that he sometimes did when I said "Down." Your dog does not have to like lying down every time you give the command. He just has to do it.

Another form of moderate resistance is what I call Floppy Dog. Floppy Dog is more annoying. It is a style of resistance, seemingly perfected by golden retrievers, in which the dog goes completely limp when you try to lift his legs and lower his body to the ground. Floppy Dog with a Twist describes the technique of rolling onto the back, waving the front legs around, and squirming around so you cannot get your hands in place. And yes, it is as exasperating as it sounds. The solution is to move the dog to a different place in the room. Get him up by lifting (if you can) or by walking forward with leash in hand, saying "Come on!" or other encouraging words. When you get him up, grasp the collar tightly and pull up slightly to avoid the Flop.

Here is what you do not want to do: let Floppy Dog stay on the ground, "since he's down there anyway." He needs to let you handle his front legs and let you lower him to the floor. Remember, this exercise is fundamentally about your pack leadership role. Don't give up on it because your dog is unwilling—or too annoying—to be handled.

Violent resistance, such as growling and biting, is a much more significant problem. As described in the previous chapter on Sit on Command, a dog that violently resists your handling may be more than you—or anyone—can handle. Read the chapters on taking charge (Chapter 7) and mouthing and biting (Chapter 10). They will give you additional information about this problem and help you decide the best response. Remember, a dog must accept being handled to be trained, and a dog must be trained to live compatibly—and safely—in your home. Do not risk harm to yourself, your spouse, your children, or your friends by living with an aggressive dog. Pets are supposed to bring us joy and companionship, not disaster.

Chapter 22

Sit-Stay

AN ADOPTED ADOLESCENT or adult dog will probably come to you with at least a few bad habits that you would like to undo. Bolting out the front door is one that I hear about frequently. Another is bounding out of the car. These behaviors may be especially strong in a dog that was once a wanderer. It may take quite a while for him to become accustomed to the confinement (and safety) of living with responsible owners. Sit-Stay will help.

Sit-Stay means that your dog must remain in a sitting position until you release him with a specific command. While he is sitting and staying he may move his head and wag his tail. He may not lie down or get up and walk away before he is released. In the beginning, this exercise should be taught and practiced in a quiet, distraction-free environment. However, our ultimate goal is that your dog will sit and stay until released even in the midst of chaos.

There are many practical uses for Sit-Stay. As mentioned above, this exercise can be used to teach your dog not to run through open doorways. It can be used as a control mechanism when you are digging through your purse or pants pocket looking for a set of car keys. Sit-Stay is a great way to keep your dog controlled while you write a check at the veterinarian's office or when you stop on the street to chat with a friend.

Sit-Stay is also the foundation for other obedience exercises, such as Come on Command and Greeting People Without Jumping. As you saw in the previous chapter, it is used in teaching Step Four of the Down on Command exercise. Mastering Sit-Stay with your dog may require diligence and practice, but the end result will be well worth your efforts.

Step One: Sitting at Your Side

* Compel your dog to sit at your left side using the Sit on Command training technique.
* While you are still bent over with your right hand through your dog's collar and your left hand on his backside, say "Stay," and stand up straight next to your dog. Do not use your dog's name prior to a Stay command.
* Keep your dog sitting and staying at your side. Gather the leash up in your right hand. Grip the leash with your left hand palm down between your right hand and your dog. Make sure that the leash is loose and that there is no tension from the leash on your dog's neck.
* Watch your dog closely. If he starts to move, growl "Nhaa!" If he stands up or lies down, bend over and slide your right hand through his collar. Using your left hand, gently haul him back to your left side and re-sit him. Repeat the command "Stay" to remind him of what he is supposed to be doing.
* Repeat this process until your dog remains sitting at your left side for twenty seconds. Your dog can move his head and wag his tail. However, he must not move out of a sitting position at your left side.
* After your dog has remained in a sitting position at your left side for twenty seconds, release him using a specific release word (see below) that means "Now you can move." After you release your dog from the stay, praise him lavishly.

Corrections for Stay

Throughout Step One of Sit-Stay, the correction for inappropriate movement is a guttural sounding "Nhaa!" It is unnecessary and counterproductive to put your dog back into position in a rough manner.

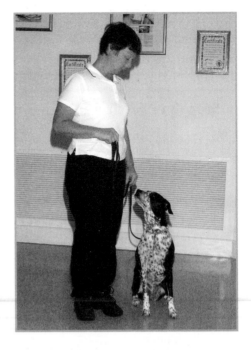

Always practice Sit-Stay with a loose leash. Quick collar corrections are only for mistakes. Be sure that at first your training environment is free of distractions.

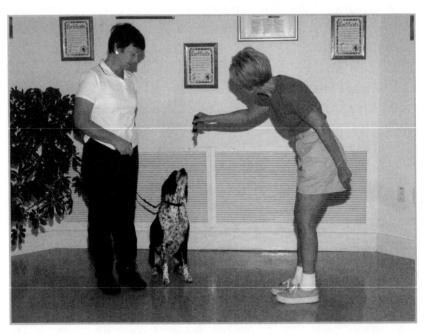

With practice, your dog will be able to sit and stay even in the presence of distractions. Teaching him to do so is called "proofing."

Replacing your dog at your left side is *not* part of the correction. When he moves from the proper Sit-Stay position, do not pounce on him. Do not drag him back to your side. Do not slam him into a sit at your side. Simply growl "Nhaa!" and then calmly and methodically replace your dog at your side.

Methodical handling is essential

All good trainers handle dogs in a calm way. Moving too quickly in a frazzled manner merely signals to your dog that you are not in control. And if your dog senses that you are not in control, he will not view you as pack leader. If you move methodically and assertively, you will carry out the training techniques more precisely and at the same time convince your dog that you are pack leader.

Release commands

I use the word "okay" to release my dog from a stay. Some trainers use the word "go" as a release word. Others use "freedom" or "release."

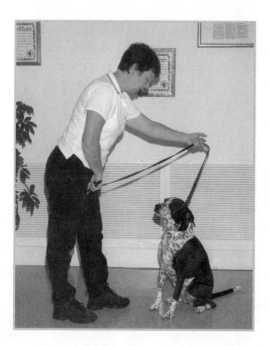

When you practice Sit-Stay in front of your dog, be sure that collar corrections are aimed back toward the dog's tail. You don't want to pull the dog forward out of position with your jerk and release.

Choose one of these or think of your own. Any word is fine as long as it has this one specific meaning to your dog: "Now you are released from a stay."

You can help your dog associate his freedom to move with your command by giving special emphasis or inflection to the command. My release word, "okay," can be lost in a sentence, such as "Is it okay if I use your car today?" Instead, I pronounce the word with a bit of zip and enthusiasm: "Ohh-kay!" It never fails to get my dog practically bouncing out of the stay with a wagging tail and ready to see what is happening next.

Doggie sit-ups

After your dog has learned to stay in a sitting position at your left side for twenty seconds, increase the time to forty seconds and then a full minute. Continue increasing the time until your dog can do a Sit-Stay at your left side for three full minutes.

I often refer to the Sit-Stay exercise as doggie sit-ups. Like sit-ups, Sit-Stay practice is both tedious and boring. Standing still for three minutes while your dog sits at your left side is comparable to watching grass grow! However, having a dog that will sit and stay reliably is essential to obedience training. In fact, a reliable Sit-Stay may arguably be more worthwhile than a flat tummy.

Stay next to your dog

Do not increase the distance away from your dog when practicing the Sit-Stay exercise at this stage of training. Practice at all times with your dog at your left side. Also, make sure that there are minimal distractions in the area that you choose for practice sessions. It is important that your dog can concentrate on you while you practice Sit-Stay Step One.

Proofing

When you are successful with Step One, you can add some distractions to the training environment. This is called proofing. Proofing means to purposely create and systematically add distractions to the training environment. These distractions may cause your dog to make a mistake so that you can correct him. Proofing is imperative in order to have a well-trained dog. Sit-Stay is worthwhile only when your dog does so reliably in the presence of distractions.

Gradual proofing

Introduce mild distractions at first. When your dog will stay successfully, increase to moderate distractions. When you are successful with moderate distractions, introduce chaotic distractions. Your goal is a dog that will stay under any circumstances.

Read your dog

Distractions are handled differently by every dog. What is considered a mild distraction by one dog may be considered a moderate or chaotic distraction by another. In the beginning, you will have to figure out what distractions are appropriate for your dog. The guideline is this: The distraction should be just enough to cause your dog to begin to get up. If you are struggling to keep your dog under control, the distraction is too intense. Back down to a moderate or mild level.

Here are some examples of distractions. Be creative in thinking of others.

* Shuffle back and forth in front of your dog.
* Whistle. (However, if you use a specific whistle to call your dog, do not use this for proofing.)
* Jingle your car keys.
* Stoop down on your dog's level.
* Have someone knock on the door or ring the doorbell.
* Clap your hands.
* Bounce a tennis ball.
* Drop a dog cookie on the floor.
* Let the cat into the room.

- ✳ Hold a dog cookie.
- ✳ Turn on the radio or TV.
- ✳ Sing a song.
- ✳ Eat a sandwich.
- ✳ Have children walk or run by.
- ✳ Have a family member clap hands near your dog's face and say his name.

The big taboo

There is one proofing taboo: Never use the command "Come." You never want to call your dog to you using the command "Come" and then correct him for responding! This would undermine all of your Come on Command training.

Step Two: Five Minutes at Left Side with Proofing

Continue to practice Sit-Stay with your dog sitting at your left side. Increase your time objective to five minutes. When you have achieved this goal, you can begin proofing your dog.

- ✳ Place your dog in a sitting position at your left side. Tell him, "Stay."
- ✳ While your dog is sitting and staying at your left side, have a friend or family member talk to your dog. He or she can say anything to your dog with the exception of the command "Come." If the command "Come" is used to proof your dog he will become inhibited to come to you when he is called.
- ✳ If your dog starts to move from the Sit-Stay position, growl "Nhaa!" Using your left hand on the leash, give a gentle jerk and release on the training collar back toward his tail.
- ✳ Gently replace your dog in a sitting position at your left side. You must be assertive if you want your dog to stay when told. However, you must never be rough while you replace your dog in the stay.
- ✳ After you replace your dog at your left side, say "Stay" to remind him of what you expect him to do.

Gradually increase the level of distractions into the training environment as your dog improves. Your goal is a five-minute Sit-Stay at your left side in the presence of many different distractions.

The big mistake

The biggest mistake that owners make when they teach their dog to stay is going too far from the dog too soon. If you say "Stay" and then walk away from your dog, you are setting yourself up for failure. When your dog moves, you will not be in position to correct him with proper timing.

Criteria for advancement

Number one: time The first concern that a good trainer should have when teaching a dog to stay is time. Ask yourself this question: Can I get my dog to stay in one place without getting up for fifteen seconds? After success with that goal, how about thirty seconds? A minute? Then two minutes, and so on, until you have reached a specific time goal. Each time increase should be no more than fifteen to twenty seconds.

Number two: distraction level of the training environment When time is no longer a factor, that is, when you think your dog will stay in place at your side for as long as you expect, you are ready for the next level of advancement. It is time to increase the distraction level in the training environment. The trainer should always start off by teaching the dog a new obedience exercise in a distraction-free setting. As the dog becomes more proficient with the stay exercise, mild distractions should be incorporated into the training environment. Continue to increase the level of distractions in the training environment as your dog becomes more reliable with the stay.

Number three: distance away from the dog When your dog will stay reliably for a designated time in a distracted environment, you can increase distance away from him. Distance should always be increased in short intervals. Three feet at a time is sufficient.

The Stay hand signal

The most common hand signal for the Stay command is an open palm placed momentarily in front of the dog's muzzle. The hand signal should be given in a deliberate manner at a normal speed. Do not flash the hand signal in front of your dog's face at lightning speed.

Step Three: Stay from in Front

* Start with your dog sitting at your left side. Place the rings of the training collar under your dog's neck. Hold the leash in your left hand by the handle. Your right hand should be free.
* Tell your dog to stay, using both the verbal command—"Stay"— and the hand signal. The hand signal for all Stay exercises is an open palm held momentarily in front of the dog's face.
* After you tell your dog to stay, take two or three steps forward, then turn and face your dog. You should be no more than halfway to the end of the leash.
* Once you are in front of your dog, grab the leash palm up with your free right hand. Your right hand will be holding the leash between your dog and your left hand.
* Watch your dog closely. If he starts to get up, growl "Nhaa!" At the same time as you growl, step toward your dog with your right leg and give a *gentle* jerk and release, back toward your dog's tail. Do not jerk toward you or straight up. Doing so will cause your dog to move from the sitting position. Only jerk in a direction that will keep your dog sitting.
* Keep your dog staying in this position for thirty seconds. At the end of thirty seconds, pivot back so that your dog is at your left side. Keep him sitting at your left side for ten seconds and then release your dog. Release him by taking a step forward as you say his release command.
* After you release your dog, praise him lavishly!

Each time you have successfully kept your dog in a Sit-Stay without having to correct him, increase the designated time by thirty seconds. Your time objective on this step is three minutes. Practice the Sit-Stay while you are standing halfway to the end of the leash.

Do not release your dog from the stay while you are still in front of him. Always return to your dog so that he is sitting at your left side before you release him. As your dog becomes reliable with the Sit-Stay while you are standing in front of him, be sure to add proofing distractions to the training environment.

Returning around your dog

An alternative to pivoting back to your dog to release him from a Sit-Stay is to return around him. This exercise is a good proofing technique. Remember that proofing teaches your dog to stay reliably in different situations.

* After you have been in front of your dog for a designated time, return to him by going to the right of him.
* Quickly go all the way around your dog without hesitating. When you are directly behind him, say "Stay." Initially, dogs often move when the handler gets to this spot. By saying "Stay" at just the right time, you will counteract his movement. All dogs are different, so you may have to adjust the spot where you say "Stay" to a slightly different position.
* After you go around your dog, stop when he is at your left side.
* Wait ten seconds and then release your dog, using the release command.
* After you release your dog, praise him lavishly.

Step Four: End of the Leash

This step is not significantly different or more difficult than Step Three. Simply walk all the way to the end of your leash and practice from this position. Be sure that as you walk away from your dog you keep your back to him at all times. Look over your shoulder at your dog to make sure that he does not move. When you reach the end of the leash, then turn and face him.

What you never want to do is back away from your dog. Backing away from your dog is part of the Come on Command training technique. Backing away after telling your dog to stay may confuse him and trigger your dog's conditioned response to come to you.

Practice the Sit-Stay exercise the same way that you did on Step Three by starting with short time increments and increasing them to longer periods. Your goal is five minutes.

Work into the environment a variety of proofing distractions. At this stage in training, contrived distractions, such as dropping your keys, probably will not faze your dog. He has seen and heard it all before, and it is likely that he will not fall for any contrived distractions.

If this is the case (which is great!), you are ready for proofing out in the world. Bring your dog to the local park or ball field to practice Sit-Stay. Do a Sit-Stay in your front yard while the neighborhood kids get off the school bus. Practice Sit-Stay on Main Street or near the entrance to the pet supply shop. Your task is to find places to train where there are natural, everyday distractions. Remember, a Sit-Stay is only as good as the dog's ability to stay in place with distractions.

Although Step Four is not significantly different or more difficult than what has come before, the next step is. Step Five will require that you go beyond the end of the leash. You will not be ready for this step until your dog does a reliable Sit-Stay while you are still holding the end of the leash. A word of caution: Be sure to practice Step Five in a dog-safe area. One mistake near a busy road could end in disaster. Don't take risks when your dog is off the leash.

Before you can go beyond the end of the leash, you must achieve two objectives. One is that your dog does a reliable Sit-Stay in the presence of distractions. The other is that when he does make a mistake, he stops dead in his tracks when you growl "Nhaa!" Until you have reached this point, continue to practice Sit-Stay by keeping the leash in your hand so that you can associate "Nhaa!" with a collar correction whenever your dog moves from the stay.

Step Five: Two Steps Beyond the End of the Leash

✳ Start with your dog sitting at your left side. Tell him to stay, using both the verbal command and the hand signal.

✳ Walk away from your dog, keeping your back to him at all times. Be sure to watch him over your shoulder as you walk away. If he starts to move, growl "Nhaa!" When you reach the end of the leash, drop it and continue on for another two feet. Then turn and face your dog.

✳ Watch your dog closely. Again, if he starts to move, growl "Nhaa!" Without the leash in your hand, perfect timing of your verbal correction is essential. You must correlate the sound "Nhaa!" with his initial movement. If your "Nhaa!" is late, your dog will not understand what you want.

✳ If the "Nhaa!" correction does not stop your dog from breaking the stay, walk calmly back to him. *Do not run back to your dog!* Running toward your dog will trigger flight instinct, and he will run away from you. Bring him back to the spot where he broke the stay and re-sit him. In a normal command tone, say "Stay."

✳ Keep your dog in a Sit-Stay for one minute. Then return to him so that he is at your left side. Wait ten seconds, then release your dog.

If your dog continues to regularly break the stay and does not stop in his tracks when you growl "Nhaa," then you are not ready to practice Sit-Stay beyond the end of the leash. Go back to the previous step and practice at six feet away from your dog with the leash in your hands.

Interestingly, you will probably find that in everyday, practical situations, you will use Sit-Stay with your dog directly at your left side. In fact, you may never find any regular use for Sit-Stay with your dog long distances from you. However, the situation may present itself where you will need to tell your dog to stay and then drop the leash and walk away. Even if these situations are rare, it pays to be prepared. And Sit-Stay at your left side with minimal distractions will always be a piece of cake if your dog masters the more challenging exercises.

Troubleshooting

Extreme squirminess can be frustrating, especially if your dog resists sitting. Go down your mental checklist regarding your dog's meals, exercise, and bathroom breaks. If his needs are satisfied, you simply have to get a little tougher. Growl "Nhaa!" when he resists your efforts to make him sit. Settle for five seconds of Sit-Stay success, if necessary, and then try for ten seconds tomorrow. With practice your dog *will* improve.

If your dog is still not comfortable being handled, refer to the troubleshooting section of Chapter 20, "Sit on Command." If handling him is not a problem, you should be able to have some success with this exercise—at least for a few moments.

Some owners do not realize that their own handling is a big distraction. Make sure that the end of your leash is not waving in the dog's face. Take off bracelets that jingle every time you move. And do not be so rough that your dog feels nervous and fidgety about receiving a harsh correction. Changing something about yourself may help your dog to have more success.

Difficulties with Sit-Stay sometimes start when you try to add distractions. It is possible that your adopted dog might have strong fears, strong habits, or an extremely shy personality. If so, choose your proofing distractions carefully. A dog that is a confirmed cat chaser or that hates other dogs might need a lot of training before he can contain himself around these distractions. A dog that is sound-sensitive may have difficulty with Sit-Stay on a noisy, urban street. Fortunately, many shy dogs gain a degree of confidence when they learn the Sit-Stay exercise. It gives them a job to do and something familiar to focus on, instead of cowering and ducking under the nearest table. See Chapter 14 for more information about shyness.

If your dog is a challenge, take your time building up his Sit-Stay abilities. Too much too soon can prevent you from having success with this exercise. Try to be content with small, steady steps toward your end result. It will help you stay motivated and will increase the odds that, eventually, your dog will master this useful exercise.

Chapter 23

Down-Stay

DOWN-STAY IS THE MOST useful and important obedience exercise that any dog—young or old—should know. In fact, if my dogs were allowed to learn one obedience command only, it would be Down-Stay. That's a strong statement! Fortunately, this skill is not hard to teach, and for most dogs it is not hard to learn.

Down-Stay means that your dog must stay in a lying-down position until released with a specific command. While doing a Down-Stay, the dog may shift position in order to get more comfortable. He may wag his tail and look around, but he is not allowed to get up. Also, I will not allow him to roll away or do "GI Joe" crawls across the room. He must stay in the down position in the designated area in which I placed him.

Why is this exercise so important? I firmly believe that the key ingredient to having a well-behaved dog is control. This does not mean drill-sergeant, overbearing, obnoxious bossiness. It means leadership and the ability to fairly and humanely direct the dog's behavior in appropriate ways.

Down-Stay is a major control obedience exercise. When your dog has this skill, you will be able to bring him into any situation with the confidence that he will behave. You certainly benefit from this, but your dog benefits even more. How? *You no longer have to isolate your dog.*

Social isolation is a significant cause of behavioral problems in dogs. Dogs that are frequently locked away feel exiled from their pack (you and your family), and all sorts of unwanted behaviors can develop. The stress of social isolation inspires dogs to bark nonstop, chew unwanted items, dig up the yard, lick themselves obsessively, become aggressive, etc., etc. These are the kinds of problems that put many dogs in the pound. No one wants to live with such problems. Furthermore, an isolated dog is not learning to behave; he is just building stronger habits of bad behaviors. A Catch-22 situation exists: The owner locks the dog away because he misbehaves, the dog misbehaves because he is locked away.

Down-Stay is the answer to this dilemma. When your dog knows how to lie down and stay, it will not be necessary to banish him when guests visit your home. Your dog will not need to be crated or put outside whenever you eat a meal. You will be able to sit comfortably in the waiting room at the veterinarian's office while your dog lies at your feet. You will be able to enjoy the pleasure and satisfaction, wherever you go, of hearing people say, "Wow! That's a great dog. My dog would never stay like that."

By teaching your dog Down-Stay, you are giving him the gift of inclusion in your life. You are teaching him a skill that allows him to be part of almost everything you do—from dinner parties to a quiet evening in front of the TV, from Little League games to backyard gardening. As I said above, if my dogs knew only one obedience exercise, it would be Down-Stay. It's that important.

Step One: Teaching Down-Stay

To be at all successful with obedience-training your dog, you must succeed with this exercise. That's because an obedient dog is one that accepts you as pack leader. If a dog will not respond to this major control exercise, it is an indication that he is challenging you.

For you to be successful teaching this exercise, you need to be persistent. If your dog gets up from the Down-Stay ten thousand times, you must put him back ten thousand times. If you give up and don't do the exercise, you are telling your dog that he is the pack leader. That is being unsuccessful!

Here's how to start:

* Pick a spot in front of your favorite chair where you would like your dog to lie down and stay.

✳ Attach your six-foot leash to your dog's collar. Give the command "Down" and then down your dog using the Step One Down on Command technique (see Chapter 21).

✳ When your dog is down, draw an imaginary circle (in your mind) around your dog. Tell him to stay, using both the verbal command—"Stay"—and the hand signal. The hand signal is an open palm placed momentarily in front of the dog's face.

✳ Have a seat in your chair. For this teaching step, you should be no more than two feet from your dog, close enough so that you can reach down and touch him.

✳ Watch him closely.

✳ Keep your dog in the down position within the imaginary circle for a full ten minutes. You may hold your leash, but be sure that it is loose. Do not restrain your dog by holding it short and tight. Or you can keep the leash stretched out in front of the dog on the floor, where you can quickly step on it if your dog attempts to bolt away.

✳ Keep an eye on your dog at all times. If he should start to move, growl "Nhaa!" as a correction. Then bend over and push him back down. Do this quickly, using minimal hand contact. However, do not slam him down! Be assertive with your dog when he breaks the Down-Stay, but do not be rough.

✳ Repeat the command "Stay" after you have corrected and replaced your dog in the down position.

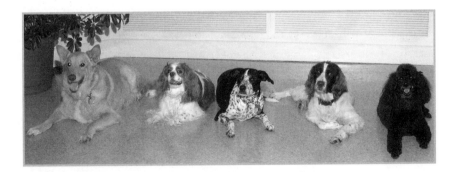

A five-dog Down-Stay. Bravo!

* The best time to correct your dog is when you feel he is thinking about getting up. Trust your intuition. If you feel he is about to get up, growl "Nhaa!" The next-best time is just as he starts to get up. The worst time is when you look up and he is gone. Watch him closely.

* At the end of ten minutes, stand up next to your dog so that he is at your left side. Hold the leash in your hands and wait ten seconds. Then release your dog by stepping forward as you say his release word, such as "Okay!"

* After you release your dog, praise him enthusiastically.

Practice this exercise for a full ten minutes every day. At first, you may only succeed in keeping your dog in the stay for a minute or even just ten to fifteen seconds. That's not a problem. Correct him when he gets up, and then put him back in place. After ten minutes of this, which may include many corrections and replacements, end the exercise with the release word and lots of praise. Practice again tomorrow and the next day. Your dog will soon get the idea of what is expected and stop getting up so often. Before you know it, he will lie there for the full ten minutes until you release him. Be sure to offer lots of praise when you do!

Step Two: Increasing Time and Distractions

A dog's Down-Stay skill is really only useful if the dog can do it in real-world situations. Step Two helps achieve that.

When your dog can lie down and stay for ten minutes without getting up, extend your practice time to twenty minutes. Eventually build up to thirty minutes. Read the newspaper if you get bored, but keep an eye on your dog. If your dog gets up, a well-timed "Nhaa!" is necessary to reinforce your training.

As we do with the Sit-Stay exercise in Chapter 22, increase distractions around your dog. Turn on the television, eat lunch, or talk on the telephone—but always be prepared to correct a mistake. As your dog's skill becomes more reliable, you also can increase the distance between you and your dog. Don't go too far at first—a few feet is plenty. Build up slowly to greater distances if you wish.

Practice outside. Use your front porch, the backyard patio, or the sidewalk in front of your house to reinforce this skill. Take your dog to the park and have him do a Down-Stay while you watch the kids play. Make him lie down and stay in the car while you pump gas. The more places you practice this exercise, the more reliably your dog will do it.

And did you notice? While you were out practicing, your dog was on an outing with you—bonding, socializing, learning to behave. In other words, being a welcomed and valued part of your life. For an adopted dog especially, that is no small thing.

Troubleshooting

Dogs that cannot relax during Down-Stay practice can be helped by having something to do. Chewing on a rawhide works great. It doesn't matter that the dog is not "paying attention" to the Down-Stay. It just matters that he does it. When your practice time is ended, release the dog with your release word, even if he is distracted with chewing. Remember, you are the one in control of the exercise.

Your dog may fall asleep while doing a Down-Stay. That's okay. A peaceful, sleeping dog is never a problem! You won't mind if he sleeps through your dinner or a TV show—as long as he stays in place. Again, when your designated time is over—even if he is sleeping—wake him up and release. And remember to praise him for staying so well.

Chapter 24

Come on Command

COME ON COMMAND is one of the most useful obedience exercises a dog can learn. It allows your dog to hang out in the backyard while you garden or play with your kids. It allows your dog to enjoy off-leash adventures in the woods, at the beach, or in a park. It can bring your dog to safety if he ever gets loose near a roadway. And it's even handy around the house when you want to round him up for a bath, clip on a leash, or practice a few obedience exercises.

Many years ago I learned a great deal about Come on Command from an adopted black standard poodle. Jossie was nineteen months old when I rescued her. She had been brought into a veterinarian's office to be "put to sleep" because the family that owned her did not have time for her.

They were not awful people. They were just too busy working and raising small children to raise and train a puppy properly. Clearly, they should never have bought a puppy in the first place. Only too late did they realize that they could not—or would not—make the time for their little canine youngster.

This family made the choice of euthanasia for Jossie because they felt that it was the only choice they had. She was nipping at their children and urinating and defecating all over their house. They had made some attempts to find a new home for her, but nobody wanted her. Considering her terrible habits, it is not hard to understand why. This family was thrilled and relieved when the veterinarian told them that I would take her.

An Adoption Challenge

When Jossie came home with me, she had every bad habit that you could think of. She understood no commands except "Sit," which most dogs manage to figure out. She jumped on people and pulled on the leash. She was not housebroken and was a destructive chewer. She would growl and nip whenever I tried to brush her or trim her toenails. And she definitely would not come when called.

Fortunately, Jossie radiated intelligence. I could tell that she was very trainable and that with proper handling she could be a great dog. And because she was only nineteen months old, her bad habits were not so deeply seated that they could not be undone.

Jossie also had a happy, fun-loving personality. She was very friendly and outgoing—not at all a fearful or grumpy creature. I felt that her nipping and growling were just bratty behaviors that she had learned to get away with in her previous home. She nipped and growled only when she was being made to do something that she did not feel like doing. Besides, she was extremely cute and gave great poodle kisses. I couldn't resist!

My experiences with Jossie make a great case study for all sorts of adoptable dog training issues. As you read about my Come on Command training efforts, you will see one (or many) of the problems that you are currently facing. If a problem dog like Jossie can overcome so many bad habits, chances are good that your dog can, too.

A week of discovery

After I had lived with Jossie for about a week, I realized that Jossie didn't just "not come" when called. She was literally conditioned to *run away* at the sound of the command "Come." Whenever I said "Jossie, come!" she would turn her body away from me and run in the opposite direction.

Intrigued by this behavior, I called her previous owners and interviewed them. I asked them precisely what they had done with Come on Command training. I was amazed by what I heard. They had made every mistake imaginable. Every technique that I teach owners to use to get their dogs to reliably run to them at the sound of the Come command these folks did in reverse. With all their mistakes, they essentially trained Jossie *not* to come!

Avoiding disagreeable experiences

One of the fundamental mistakes that Jossie's owners made was to make coming to them a disagreeable experience. Keep in mind that one of the most fundamental ways in which dogs learn is by avoiding unpleasant experiences. If dogs do a behavior and the results are disagreeable, they will learn to avoid doing that behavior.

This is what Jossie's previous owners did. They would find Jossie with a shoe, a child's toy, or some other inappropriate item in her mouth. They would call her to them, and then when she reached them, they reprimanded her for having the item. In their minds, they thought that they were teaching Jossie to leave the forbidden items alone. Instead, Jossie was associating the punishment with coming to her owners. After several experiences she stopped coming. Demanding "Come here right now!" in a harsh tone of voice didn't help. Neither did chasing after her. Here's why.

Vocal communication

Using harsh tones when calling a dog is a common mistake that many owners make. In Jossie's case, it only compounded her owners' problems. They would call her and when she did not respond immediately, they would start yelling at her. She was certainly smart enough to avoid coming toward that!

The lesson here is to use a pleasant, inviting tone of voice whenever you call your dog. If you use a harsh tone the dog will probably run away—or soon learn to. This is because a threatening or frightening tone triggers a self-preservation response in dogs, called flight instinct. If dogs do not feel that running away is an option, they will submit. They will do this by standing and cowering or lying down and rolling belly up.

Body posture, a primary canine language

Your threatening body posture will also trigger flight instinct or a submissive response. A person who is screaming and yelling will almost always have a threatening body posture. Jossie came to associate the command "Come" with a personal threat to her safety. She was a smart and perceptive puppy. She was not going to run into the mouth of the lion! Her instincts said, "Stay away," and she did.

Catch me if you can

Jossie's owners chased after her in an attempt to catch her when she would not come to them. Actually, they did successfully catch her one time. They told me that they "really gave it to her!" when they caught her. They said that they did not hurt her, just lightly whapped her on the backside as they told her she was a bad dog and then dragged her into the house.

Unfortunately for these owners, their attempts at teaching Jossie backfired. By chasing Jossie and then using misguided discipline, all that the dog learned was to be *sure* to run away at the sound of the command "Come."

Conditioned response

A dog that comes reliably when called has a conditioned response to the command "Come!" A conditioned response is a learned behavior that is automatically triggered by a cue. To develop a conditioned response, you first have to find a way to get your dog to do the behavior. Then you have to associate a command (cue) with the behavior. You must then consistently repeat the behavior and the command to form an association. After enough repetition, all you need to do is give the command and the dog will perform the behavior.

Practice makes perfect

After months of calling "Jossie, come!" in angry, threatening tones—coupled with an "I'd like to ring your neck" body stance plus futile attempts to run after and catch her—the owners gave up.

But by this time a conditioned response had developed. The cue was the command "Come." Jossie's learned behavior was to run away. As soon as she heard the command "Come," she automatically moved away from whoever was saying it.

A better way: the chase reflex

Dogs chase things that move quickly. It is called the chase reflex. It is an instinct carried over from their wild canine cousins that hunt for survival. Running down jackrabbits and caribou is the way that wolves and coyotes catch supper.

You have probably heard the warning that if a dog comes barking aggressively at you, do not run. Running will cause a dog in an aggressive state to chase and bite. Most dogs leave cats alone—until the kitty decides to run. Then the chase begins.

Chase reflex in training

Many dog trainers capitalize on the dog's chase reflex in training. The chase aspect of hunting is channeled into the skills that herding dogs use to move sheep and cattle. Guard dogs are stimulated to attack by human "agitators" who run from them. I use the chase reflex in my obedience-training program to get puppies to run to me.

If you squat down on your puppy's level and use a pleasant, friendly tone when you call his name and the command "Come," chances are good that he will come running to you. If he is busy sniffing around and does not come immediately, stand up and repeat the "Come" command and then run away from him. Running away will trigger his chase reflex, and he will run after you. When you see him chasing you, squat down, clap your hands, and verbally encourage him to come to you using pleasant tones. There! You found a way to get a puppy to do the behavior that you want. With practice (and the help of specific training techniques), this will eventually become a conditioned response.

Practicing not coming

Because I knew Jossie would not come when called, I was careful not to take her off the leash. I did not want to continue the pattern of *not* coming. Getting into a situation where I was saying "Jossie, come! Jossie, come!" and she was ignoring me would only reinforce her unwanted habit of not coming.

To complicate my Come on Command training efforts, another of Jossie's bad habits was shooting out of open doorways. The first week that I had her she succeeded in doing this a few times. After three or four escapes, I "tightened up the ship" and made sure that she was secured before the front door was opened. However, I learned something else during her few flights of freedom.

Jossie would get outside and then race up and down the sidewalk. Needless to say, she did not come to me when I called her. As a matter of fact, this was where I discovered that "Jossie, come!" made her run farther away from me. I discovered that she was so distrustful in this situation that even pleasant verbal tones and nonthreatening body stances were not enough to get her to come. I knew that she liked doggie treats, too, but they were not working in this situation.

A secret weapon?

Jossie loved my German shorthaired pointer, Jena. They became great friends from the moment they met. So the first time Jossie ran out the door, I went into the house and got Jena. I hoped that Jossie would come if Jena was with me. She did seem interested and came closer. However, as soon as I said, "Jossie, come!" she took off.

Praise, doggie treats, and a Ford F-100

I did not know how to get this frustrating dog back into the house. I decided to try to approach her calmly and see if I could get ahold of her. Before I started toward Jossie, I put Jena into the enclosed back of my old pickup truck, which was sitting in the driveway.

I opened the truck tailgate and told Jena to "kennel up," which was her command to get in. Before I could turn around, Jossie had hopped into the back of the truck with Jena! I gave her a doggie treat, praised her lavishly, and gave her lots of kisses.

The next time Jossie got out, I tried the truck technique, and sure enough, she came running and jumped in. She apparently had a pleasant association with going in the car. From then on, whenever Jossie got out, I used the truck to call her back. I made sure that she got a doggie treat and lots of praise. At last I had found a way to get her to do the behavior that I wanted. This is always step one in any training effort.

How I tired out an energetic poodle

Partly because of Jena, I was able to exercise Jossie by taking her on hiking adventures. The fact that she was not yet trained to come when called was not an issue on our hikes for a couple of reasons. For one, Jossie was the type of dog who stuck close to the pack. Also, I never took her hiking in an area where she might get in the way of a car. Driving to some wilderness trails about an hour from my home was part of our weekly activities.

Follow the pack

Along with Jena, the German shorthaired pointer, I also owned a big red Irish setter named Jason. Wherever Jena and Jason went, Jossie followed. Fortunately, Jason and Jena were both well-trained dogs that dependably came when called. During our hikes, I would call them in periodically, and Jossie would come racing along, too. When they reached me I would make everyone sit and then reward each of them with lots of praise and a doggie treat. At the end of the hike, I would open the tailgate of my pickup truck and command the dogs to "kennel up." All three dogs would leap into the truck.

Our hikes were very beneficial to the pack bonding process. Moving as a pack through the fields and woods helped Jossie feel that she was a part of the group. She would hear me call the other dogs, and she would see them come running to me. Jossie would follow and, by doing so, began to view me as pack leader. The warm reception that she received when she reached me, along with sharing some food, helped her learn to trust me. If a dog trusts you, he will try to do anything within his capability to please you. Remember: Dogs only want to please their pack leaders.

Group therapy

Even when we were at home, I took advantage of Jossie's willingness to follow the group. I would sit on the floor with my back against a wall. I would call the dogs using a happy, enthusiastic tone of voice, and they would all come running. I would give them some little treats while I praised and petted them. The dogs loved this! They would climb all over me, licking and nuzzling my body. It had a very wolfy feel, a real 1970s love fest.

In my fenced backyard, Jossie was sometimes reluctant to come when called if she was out there by herself. When I called her she would just stand there and stare at me. I did not repeat the command, because I wanted to avoid practicing "not coming." I simply turned and walked into the house. Ten seconds later there she would be, standing at the back door wagging her tail. I would praise her warmly and let her in. Of course, if she was with the other dogs, she always followed them right in when I called.

All good things come with time

During the first six weeks with me, Jossie made great strides. I spent a lot of time handling her. I brushed her every day. I cleaned her ears twice a week. I handled her feet, mouth, and legs on a regular basis. Initially she did not like the intrusion. She tried her growling and snapping routine. When she did this I was firm but never rough in correcting her. Each and every time I would growl "Nhaa!" using a firm and guttural tone. Before long, her aggressive behavior was a thing of the past.

By the second week Jossie would tolerate being handled without growling, but she still was apprehensive. After a few more weeks of daily handling she actually seemed to like it, except for ear cleaning and toenail trimming. She never came to enjoy these two doggie maintenance procedures, but she would stoically accept having them done.

After about six weeks of doing everything described here, Jossie had come a long way in learning to trust me. She was definitely my little curly girlfriend, and I felt (at last!) that she was ready for formal training. Here is how we started Come on Command.

Golden Rules for Come on Command

I took essentially the same approach to training Jossie to come on command as I had with Jason and Jena. First, I made sure that I was aware at all times of the factors that influence coming reliably. Here is a checklist of things to remember.

* Be aware of your vocal tone and body language. Never sound and look as if you are a threatening creature. Squat down on your dog's level, and call him using a friendly, exuberant tone of voice.

* Make sure that coming to you always results in an agreeable experience for your dog. Remember, dogs avoid unpleasant experiences. If you correct your dog when he reaches you, he will learn to avoid you.

* Never chase your dog. If you run after your dog you will trigger his flight instinct, and he will run away from you. The only thing that you will teach your dog is that he can outrun you. If your dog does not come when you call, run *away* from him to trigger his chase reflex.

* Do not let your dog practice ignoring your Come command. Repeatedly calling your dog while he ignores you (or runs away from you) is teaching him to ignore the command. If you practice this every day, you will end up with a dog that is well trained to ignore the Come command.

Exercising a Dog That Will Not Come

When I got my springer spaniel, Crea, she was eight weeks old. I was living year-round on Nantucket Island, which is off the coast of Cape Cod in Massachusetts. Our house was on a pond, with a long backyard covered with pine trees.

Because Crea was young and in a brand-new environment, she stuck very close to me during her first few days in the backyard. As a matter of fact, I remember one time accidentally stepping on one of her little paws because she was so underfoot. But each day she became progressively more confident and brave. By the end of the first week she was boldly poking around the yard exploring. Still, she would only go maybe forty feet from me.

When she was a short distance from me, I would frequently squat down on her level, call "Crea, come!" in an enthusiastic tone, and wave her tennis ball. She always came running to me as fast as she could. I would lure her close with the tennis ball and praise her lavishly when she came to me.

Each week Crea's confidence grew. By the time she was four months old, she would independently explore the entire yard. Yet no matter how far from me she ventured, she always came running when I squatted down and called "Crea, come!" That is, until one morning.

It was a morning just like all the others. We were in the backyard, and she was nosing around. She got right to the edge of my property, near an empty lot, and was sniffing something that she seemed to find highly interesting. I squatted and called "Crea, come!" She looked over at me, and I showed her the tennis ball. She went right back to sniffing.

I do not like to repeat commands, but I did. I called her name and "Come" again. She ignored me. I stood up and very calmly and nonchalantly approached her. I knew not to rush toward her, because I did not want to frighten her and trigger her flight instinct. Despite this, when she looked up and saw me moving toward her, she beelined it through the empty lot and down along the pond.

Now, human nature being what it is, this is when most owners get angry and begin yelling and chasing after their "disobedient" dog. And heaven help the dog when he is captured. A verbal scolding (or worse) is often the punishment for "not coming when I called you!"

There's a better way, which produces much better results. I did not chase Crea. I knew that she was in a safe area away from the road, and I felt confident that she would not go too far. So I walked back to the house to get her leash and a couple of doggie treats. I returned to find Crea three or four properties down the pond. She was busy eating Canada goose poops and did not seem to mind my approach. I clipped her leash on and walked her home. When I got back to the house and told Barbara what had happened, she said, "Time for the long line." She was absolutely right.

The long line—your "upper hand"

A long line is a thirty-foot piece of yellow nylon rope with a dog leash clip woven onto one end. I kept mine on the deck by the back door. The next time I took Crea to the backyard, I clipped the long line to her buckle collar.

After about ten minutes in the yard, Crea wandered over to the same area she had been so interested in that morning. I squatted and called "Crea, come!" Just as before, she looked up at me and then went back to sniffing. This time, however, I did not go toward Crea. I looked for the end of the long line, walked over to it, and stepped on it. Then I picked up the long line and, watching Crea, ran for the house. When all of the slack ran out of the long line, Crea was nudged in my direction. I did not flip her over or send her flying. She just received a little tug.

When Crea felt this and saw me running away from her, she came chasing after me. I then squatted down, verbally encouraged her to come over to me, and when she reached me, I praised her lavishly. I then walked her into the house.

The long line was my upper hand. It gave me the ability to call Crea *once* and make her come to me. Without the long line, Crea would have had the upper hand. I would have been in a position, day after day, of calling her and not getting the appropriate response. Crea quickly would have learned that "Come!" meant to ignore me and to keep on exploring (or eating goose poops).

When I described this experience to Barbara, I remember saying, "The long line worked great. But Crea is such a ball of fire that she will probably be dragging it for the next seven years." But I was wrong.

I used the long line consistently with Crea. I put it to use whenever we went on dog hikes on the beaches and moors of Nantucket. In fact, I attached the long line any time I removed Crea's training leash and I was not 100 percent certain that she would respond immediately when called.

Along with using the long line, I was careful not to make mistakes that would undermine my Come on Command training objectives. I practiced the on-leash chase reflex training exercises with Crea almost every day. By the time Crea was one year old, she had developed such a strong conditioned response to the command "Come" that I no longer needed the long line. She responded to my call almost every time.

Almost? Yes, because no learned behavior is infallible. Even the best-trained dogs can make mistakes. Never take any dog off the leash near a roadway or other dangers. One small slip-up could have disastrous results.

On-Leash Chase Reflex Training Exercises

In order to train your dog to come when called reliably, you must teach him what you want. Here are two techniques that you should practice with your dog every day.

First technique: chase reflex

This technique and the following one capitalize on your dog's instinctive chase reflex. The chase reflex makes dogs follow after things that quickly move away from them.

Dogs also have a flight instinct in which they run away from things that chase after *them*. Rule number one is never to call your dog to you and then chase after him if he does not respond. Doing so would eventually condition him to run away when he hears the command "Come."

If your dog does not come when called, you run away from him.

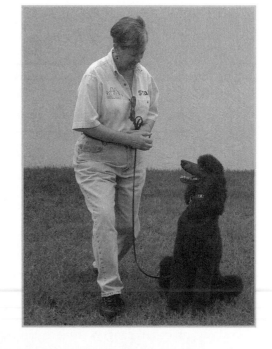

Come on Command training begins with a simple chase reflex. With your dog sitting at your side, step off backward and say "Come!" Reward your dog warmly when he turns to follow you.

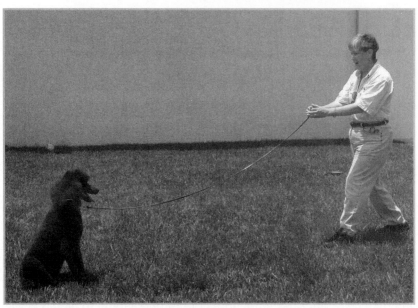

Practice Come on Command a few feet away from your dog. Say "Come!" as you step off backward. Give him lots of praise and hugs when he comes running to you.

This will trigger his chase reflex and he will come running after you. When he does start moving in your direction, squat down on his level and praise him until he reaches you. Then pet and praise him lavishly. Remember: Never correct your dog when he comes to you!

* Start with your dog sitting at your left side. Say, "Stay." Hold the leash with both hands, one directly above the other. The leash should be as loose as possible without wrapping around your dog's legs.
* Call your dog's name, followed by the command "Come." Hesitate two seconds, then run backward away from your dog. You do not have to be a track star to do this exercise effectively. Back up at whatever speed you are comfortable with.
* If your dog does not follow after you when you run away from him, give a gentle jerk and release on the collar. Jerk gently—do not flip your dog over backward.
* If en route to you your dog becomes distracted and veers off in another direction, give a gentle jerk and release on the collar. The leash should never be tight. It should always be slack, unless you are jerking and releasing. Do not reel him in like a fish.
* Praise your dog enthusiastically as he is moving toward you.
* When your dog reaches you, gently tuck him into a sit. Praise him warmly! Make him think this is the best thing he has ever done.

Be sure that your command is clear and pleasant. For best results, practice this Come on Command exercise twelve times a day. And do not undo your hard work by practicing *not* coming.

Second technique: chase reflex from six feet away

For this step to be effective your dog must be able to do a Sit-Stay (see Chapter 22).

* Start with your dog sitting at your left side. Hold the leash by the handle in your left hand.

How to Use a Long Line

A long line is twenty-five to fifty feet of rope or cord clipped to the dog's buckle collar. The long line gives you the upper hand for getting your dog back whenever you take him off the leash. Without a long line, an unleashed dog has the upper hand. If he does not feel like coming when called, all you can do is stand there *practicing not coming* by repeating the Come command without getting the right response.

When your dog is clipped to a long line, you call your dog once. If he does not respond, don't worry about what the dog is doing. Look for the end of the long line. Walk over to it, step on it, then pick it up. (Never pick up a moving rope. You might get a painful rope burn.)

When you have the long line in hand, move quickly in the opposite direction away from your dog. This will trigger the chase reflex and cause your dog to come running after you. If your dog is not paying attention to you (sniffing a bush, etc.), he may get tugged in your direction. Make sure that you do not flip him over. A gentle nudge will do the trick. Also, be careful that the long line is not wrapped around his legs.

As your dog is running toward you, squat down on his level and wave his favorite object of attraction (tennis ball, treat, etc.) to get his attention. Verbally encourage him to you. Hold the object of attraction out in front of you so that your dog does not run past you. When he reaches you, give him lots of praise and hugs. Make him think that coming when called is the best thing he has ever done!

The long line enables you to keep your dog coming to you while you work with Come on Command obedience training. Your goal is to form a solid habit in your dog of coming every time he is called. To be successful with this, be sure to use the long line every time you take your dog off the leash. Do not make the common mistakes described in Jossie's story. And practice vigorously the on-leash training steps described here.

* Use both the verbal command and the hand signal, tell your dog, "Stay." As you walk away from your dog, keep your back to him but look over your shoulder at him. Walk to the end of the leash, and then continue on until you are one arm length beyond the end of the leash.

* When your left arm is stretched behind you, turn and face your dog. Hold the leash in both hands about chest level. Both arms should be stretched out toward your dog. The leash should not be slack, but it should not be completely tight. Hold the leash at the point just before it would become tight.

* In a clear voice, call your dog's name followed by the command "Come." A second after you give the command, give a gentle jerk and release on the collar and run backward away from your dog. Keep facing your dog as you run away from him.

* Be sure to praise your dog as he moves toward you. Keep the leash loose as he moves toward you. Do not reel or pull him in like a fish.

* Use his favorite object of attraction to lure him to you. Do not let him run by you. When your dog reaches you, lure him into the sitting position with the object of attraction. If he does not follow the object into a sitting position, gently compel him to sit.

* After he is sitting, tell him, "Stay." Praise and pet your dog. Do not let him pop up. Pivot back so that your dog is sitting at your left side. Wait ten seconds, and then either release him or do another repetition of the exercise.

You should practice twelve repetitions of each chase-reflex technique with your dog every day. If you want a dog that comes reliably when you call him, you must develop a conditioned response.

Reinforcing the stay

Practice this variation of the second technique. After you have reached the end of the leash and have turned to face your dog, hold the leash as if you were going to call him. However, instead of calling your dog, walk back to him. As you approach your dog, praise him and remind him, "Stay." Go directly to him. Stand in front of him, nose to knees.

Give your dog a small food reward for staying. As you do this, praise him lavishly, but do not let him break the stay. Now pivot back so that your dog is sitting at your left side. Then either release him or leave him to do another Come on Command. By returning to your dog periodically—as opposed to calling him every time you reach the end of the leash—you will prevent him from anticipating the command before you give it. It will make your dog even more attentive to the command.

Troubleshooting

My experiences with Jossie, described above, will give you a good idea of the many problems you may have with this exercise. Creating and strengthening a bond with your adopted dog is an important part of overcoming some of these problems. So is keeping your dog under your control by using a long line.

One of the more difficult problems you may have is an adopted dog that is a former street waif. Such a dog, especially an adult one, has strong habits of taking off and wandering for hours or days or weeks at a time. Many are unneutered males, following their hormonal urges around town. The street waif has little or no experience with being bonded to a human owner or with obeying any commands. Anytime you unclip this dog's leash, he's off like a rocket headed for the next county. He has no interest in hanging around with you.

Your best bet with this dog is to keep him under your control at all times—and if appropriate, get him neutered. Be sure you have an escape-proof backyard, are vigilant by the front door, and have a sturdy leash for plenty of on-leash exercising. This dog has a long way to go before he will learn Come on Command. Which does not mean that he will never respond. Depending on the dog's age, personality, and previous experiences, he may learn to bond with you, enjoy the praise and rewards of Come on Command training, and quickly adapt to the new behaviors you are teaching. But until then, keep him safe and secure. His urge to roam far and wide, never responding to your call, will be strong unless you take steps to turn it around.

Postscript

Just a last word about Jossie: She overcame virtually all of her bad habits. Along with earning two American Kennel Club obedience titles, she turned out to be one of the best dogs that I have ever owned. Never underestimate an adopted dog!

Chapter 25

Walking on a Leash

ALMOST EVERY DOG needs to know how to walk properly on a leash. If you live in a city, your dog will probably walk on a leash several times a day to eliminate plus enjoy outings for exercise, trips to the veterinarian, and visits to see friends. Suburban and country dogs may have daily leash walks for exercise, or they may be clipped to a leash going to or from the car, into the vet's office, or across the parking lot leaving the groomers.

If your adopted dog drags you along on the leash, going out together will, literally, be a drag. You won't enjoy it, the dog probably won't enjoy it, and soon you won't be doing it very much at all.

If outings with your dog dwindle to almost nothing, you soon will have an unexercised, unsocialized dog that is bored and stuck in the house. That's a perfect formula for all sorts of trouble—housebreaking mistakes, destructive chewing, excessive barking, stress-induced health problems, aggression, shyness, etc. I cannot emphasize enough that getting out and about with your dog is essential to his well-being. An important way to make sure that happens is to teach him good leash-walking skills.

My definition of a dog that has good leash skills is a dog that can walk on a loose leash without pulling and that keeps his attention focused on you, the handler. I call it Controlled Walking. Controlled Walking is not heeling, which requires a dog to stay directly at the handler's left side, adjusting precisely to whatever speed and direction the handler moves.

Controlled Walking is a little looser, and it is perfect for pets. It allows you and your dog to walk comfortably down the street without the dog gagging against his collar and you having an arm pulled out of your shoulder socket. It allows your dog to see cats and squirrels without lunging wildly, it allows you to stop and chat with a friend without canine disturbance, and it allows you and your dog to jog or run if you want more strenuous exercise. Again, the dog's job is to stay with you on a loose leash and to be attentive to your movements. If you have never walked a dog that has this skill, I can guarantee that you are in for a pleasant surprise.

The Preliminary: Controlled Standing

The first step in teaching good leash-walking skills is to teach good leash-*standing* skills. There's no sense in moving if your dog cannot even behave while you are standing still. Here's how to start:

* Hold the leash in your right hand, with your left hand directly below it. Keep both hands together. Allow the leash to be as loose as possible without it touching the ground or wrapping around your dog's legs.
* Draw an imaginary circle around your body. This is the area in which your dog is expected to remain while you are standing still. The edge of the circle should be about three feet from you. Your dog should be kept in this circle on a loose leash at all times.
* When your dog attempts to move out of the circle, give a jerk and release on the collar. The correction should be directed toward your body. Do not pull your dog back to you. Always jerk and release. Jerk and release until your dog is back inside your imaginary circle. When he is inside the circle, stop jerking immediately and praise your dog.

Jerks and releases do not have to be given in a hard or harsh manner in order to be effective. Start with a gentle jerk and release. If your

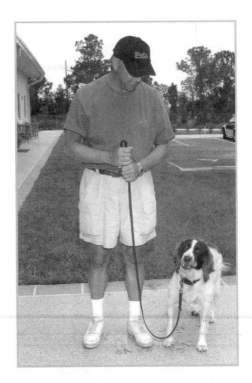

Controlled Standing is a prerequisite to good leash-walking skills. There's no sense trying to move forward on a loose leash until your dog can manage doing so just standing still.

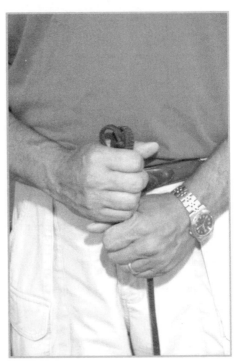

Grip the leash with one hand above the other for this exercise. Note that the end of the leash is folded up so that it does not distract the dog.

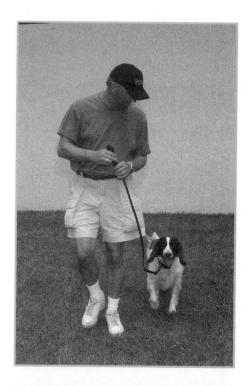

Step off with your dog. Move forward at a steady pace but keep your eyes on your dog.

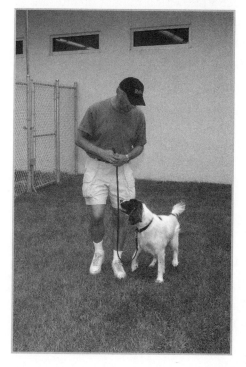

Without tipping off the dog with a verbal command or body gesture, back up in your tracks to your starting position. An attentive dog will be aware of your movement and turn his body to follow you. Praise the dog warmly when he does this! He is learning Controlled Walking.

dog is unresponsive, jerk a little harder. It will not take long before you find the proper amount of force required to teach your dog to stop pulling.

Your dog will quickly learn that it is *agreeable* to stay comfortably by your side on a loose leash. He will learn that it is *dis*agreeable to pull or lunge away from you, because it always results in a correction. The more consistent you are with your handling (keeping a loose leash inside the circle, giving a jerk and release whenever the dog goes beyond it), the quicker your dog will understand what to do. With practice you will be able to stand still in any environment and have your dog under control on a loose leash.

As with other training exercises, it is important that you begin teaching Controlled Standing in a good training environment. Keep distractions to a minimum at first. As your dog improves, increase the distractions. For example, turn on the TV or let the kids into the room. Let the cat walk by. Try going outside to practice Controlled Standing. Chat with your neighbor or look in a shop window.

It is okay to praise your dog when he stays near you on a loose leash, especially when you see him notice a distraction but not pull toward it. Correct him with a quick jerk and release if he makes a mistake and starts to lunge or pull. With each well-timed correction, you are one step closer to improving your dog's reliability with this exercise.

Step One: Walking on a Loose Leash

Remember that Controlled Walking has two objectives. The first is to walk on a loose leash without ever pulling. The second is to be constantly attuned to the handler at the other end of the leash. Step One focuses on the first objective: no pulling!

* Start with your dog at your left side. Hold the leash with both hands together, the same way you did with Controlled Standing. Make sure that the leash is not tight. There should be a large loop in the leash between your hands and your dog.
* Walk forward with your dog at a normal brisk pace. Your dog does not have to stay on your left side while walking. (This is not heel-

ing.) If he goes to your right side, simply switch the leash around your body. You must keep an eye on your dog the entire time you are teaching Controlled Walking so that you know where he is.

✳ When you anticipate that your dog is about to pull, slide your left hand midway down the leash and give a quick jerk and release. Do *not* growl "Nhaa!" at your dog as you jerk and release. Let the collar give the correction.

✳ After you jerk and release, slide your left hand back up under your right hand, so that both hands are together again.

✳ When your dog is not pulling and the loop is in the leash, praise your dog, using a calm, pleasant voice.

The main thing a handler must do in order to be successful teaching Controlled Walking is to adopt a simple mind-set: loose leash at all times or jerk and release. This means that the handler never allows the leash to become tight. You must be relentless with yourself in order to be successful. If you are inconsistent and sometimes allow your dog to pull on the leash, you will undermine your training. Remember: loose leash at all times. Jerk and release before the leash becomes tight.

Proper corrections

A training collar only becomes a choke collar when you allow the dog to pull on the leash or if you purposely constrict the collar around the dog's throat. Choking your dog can cause injury. This is not our goal!

Besides hurting your dog, choking teaches him nothing—except to be fearful of the individual who is choking him. Jerking and releasing on a training collar in the proper way gives a correction that will not cause harm. You do not need to jerk and release violently.

Not only are violent corrections unnecessary for successful training, they are also counterproductive. When dogs are being hurt, they are out of emotional control. Dogs cannot learn when they are in this mental state. Effective corrections are bothersome to the dog, enough so that they want to avoid them, but they are not painful.

There are three ways of jerking and releasing a training collar, but only one way is the correct way. One incorrect way is called an under-correction. This means that you are not jerking hard enough and as a result your dog is ignoring you. Jerk a little harder.

Another incorrect way is an overcorrection. This means you jerked on the collar too hard and your dog yipped in pain. You hurt him! Dogs should never yip in pain with a collar correction. Don't jerk as hard the next time. The jerk and release should cause your dog to respond without hurting him.

There is no set formula for how hard to jerk and release, because all dogs are different. What might be too hard for one dog may not be hard enough for another. To find what is best for your dog, start off easy. If he does not respond, jerk a little harder. If you accidentally make him yip, back off a bit. You will find the right formula for your dog.

How to hold the leash

The most difficult aspect of Controlled Walking for the handler to master is holding the leash without allowing the leash to get tight. Whenever your dog is not pulling, you should hold the leash with both hands together. Your right hand should be on top of your left hand. Your hands should be held at waist level. The leash should be as loose as it can be without wrapping around your dog's legs.

Your left hand is mobile. If your dog starts to forge ahead, to the side, or behind you, immediately slide your left hand about midway down the leash and give a quick jerk and release. This will inhibit your dog from pulling to the end of the leash. After jerking and releasing, immediately slide your left hand back up the leash so that both hands are together again. This takes a little practice. Keep in mind that techniques work only as well as they are performed. If you master this technique, you will be rewarded with good response from your dog.

Step Two: Paying Attention

Your dog's eyes do not have to be glued to yours for this exercise. In fact, your dog does not really have to be looking at you at all. But he has to be paying attention. Dogs have better peripheral vision than humans do. They can be watching us "out of the corner of their eye."

They also have great hearing and may be listening to the volume and speed of our footsteps. And they can certainly smell us, much better than we can measure. All of these senses will help your dog pay attention to you during Controlled Walking.

Remember that half the fun of this skill is enjoying outdoor time with your dog. Your dog can and should be looking around, watching people, animals, trees, cars, bicycles, etc. Fortunately, he can learn to do all of these things and still pay attention to you at the other end of the leash.

* Start in an area with minimal distractions.
* Hold the leash in your right hand, with your left hand directly below it. Keep both hands together throughout the entire exercise. Allow the leash to be as loose as possible without it touching the ground or wrapping around your dog's legs.
* Pick a destination about twenty feet away. Look at your dog and step off toward that destination. Walk at a normal, brisk pace.
* As you are about halfway to your destination, smoothly back up in your tracks. Do not turn your body away from your dog. Do not run backward as we do with the Come on Command chase reflex exercises. Merely back up at the same speed that you were moving forward. Keep your eyes on your dog at all times so that you do not trip over him.
* If your dog keeps moving forward as you back up, give a jerk and release on the training collar with the leash. Do not pull on the leash or reel in the dog like a fish on a line. Just a quick jerk and release.
* After you have given a jerk and release, your dog will turn to look at you. As soon as he looks at you, praise him enthusiastically! Continue praising your dog while you move backward until you reach your original starting spot. When your dog reaches you, pet and praise him some more.
* If your dog turns to look at you as soon as you back up, do *not* jerk him. The jerk on the collar *only* comes if he is not paying attention to you. If he is paying attention, he will notice that you have changed direction and will turn his head to see what you are doing. Praise your dog when he does this!

- ✳ Continue praising as you back up to your original starting spot, encouraging your dog to follow.
- ✳ Step off again, repeating the walking-forward-then-backing-up process.
- ✳ Practice many times, until your dog turns and looks at you without having to be jerked. Your goal is four successful repetitions.

If you are consistent with your handling, your dog will learn to be mentally focused on you at all times. This is not foolproof, however. Distractions will make it harder for your dog to pay attention to you. As before, practice at first in areas of minimal distractions. Then step up to moderate. Remember that dogs handle distractions differently. What may bore one dog will make another dog wild. Choose distractions that are appropriate to your dog's level of "distractibility" and training.

Lifetime Reinforcement

Although I have not competed in obedience trials for many, many years, I still have well-trained dogs. They are my pets and family members. Yet despite being trained by a professional obedience instructor, they are not perfect. Like me, they make mistakes. Any intense distraction can make them forget what they are supposed to be doing.

Throughout his life, your dog will need a correction from time to time while doing Controlled Walking. A squirrel running across the sidewalk, a loose dog in someone's yard, a bicycle whizzing by—these sorts of things may inspire your dog to start pulling at the leash. Rather than yell and drag your dog away, simply back up, jerking and releasing as you go. Let the training collar do the correcting, as always. When your dog turns in your direction, stop the jerks and praise him! Ignoring a big distraction is a big accomplishment, even for a well-trained dog.

I sometimes will see a distraction before my dog does, or I will sense that my dog is in a general state of being inattentive. That's when I back up, too. Sometimes I catch him ignoring me, sometimes not.

Leash Walking Propaganda

Criticism of fundamental training methods has appeared from time to time over the past decade. This is particularly true with training techniques designed to teach leash-walking skills.

Some trainers recommend head halters for this purpose. They claim to have concerns about choking dogs or torturing them with pinch collars. As described in Chapter 18, "Using the Right Equipment," a head halter is not a training tool. It is a restraint mechanism. It works by allowing the handler to pull the dog's head in any given direction. Where the head goes, the animal will follow.

Keep in mind that techniques that involve pulling or restraint teach dogs nothing. If you want a dog that understands how to walk on a leash without pulling, you will need to use effective training tools and learn to use them correctly. You will also need to teach your dog the Controlled Walking exercise. Fortunately, these goals are not difficult to achieve with the help of a good training program.

I believe that trainers who truly think that a training collar cannot be used without choking a dog must be inept. Those who think a pinch collar is cruel when used properly on the appropriate dog must be ignorant. And those who think it is too difficult for most dog owners to learn to use these training tools properly and to master the Controlled Walking training techniques must be poor obedience instructors.

My students and their dogs do great with the Controlled Walking exercise. They are able to give fair and well-timed corrections, they encourage their dogs with enthusiastic praise, and they quickly learn the Controlled Walking training techniques. As a result, they have dogs with great leash-walking skills. They have the skills to reinforce good leash behavior at any time, either during training or later in the dog's life. They do not need to rely on a special halter or other contraption for their dog to behave. Instead, they have a well-trained dog.

Remember, the collar correction only comes when he is not tuned in and continues ahead while you are backing up. But if he turns and looks at you when you back up, he gets praise as a reward for paying attention—and no jerks. With a trained dog it only takes one little reminder like this to bring up his attention level. Then you can proceed with your walk with ease.

Troubleshooting

An adopted dog that has never worn a collar or been clipped to a leash will not be ready for this exercise, but with a little help from you he can soon begin learning it. I would handle such a dog in the same way that I handle little puppies, by introducing them properly to a leash and collar. In my book *Puppy Preschool*, I describe proper introduction to the leash by suggesting that owners clip the leash to a buckle collar and let the dog drag it around the house or yard. Careful supervision is required so that the leash does not wrap around furniture, bushes, etc.

If your adopted dog is nervous about being handled, even to let you clip on the leash, work on handling skills for a while. Buckle and unbuckle his collar a few times each day. Brush him, look at his teeth, trim his toenails. Attach the leash to his collar and then immediately unclip it. Let your dog get used to the sounds and sensations of this very basic aspect of being someone's pet.

After a few days of dragging the leash around, pick up the end of the leash and follow the dog. Go where he wants to go. Try to keep the leash loose, as you do *not* want to encourage pulling. Next, hold an object of attraction in one hand while you encourage the dog to go in your direction. Praise your dog when he moves with you. With a little practice, wearing a leash and collar will be no big deal, and you can start with the training steps described in this chapter.

At the other end of the spectrum is the dog that couldn't care less about the leash and collar. This dog is bouncing off the end of the leash at every other moment, jumping on the handler, or rolling on the floor in a Floppy Dog protest (see Chapter 23). This dog needs some settling down before most handlers can manage some success with leash walking. My efforts with such a dog would be focused on a few obedience basics, such as Sit on Command, Down on Command, and Sit-Stay. By learning these basic skills, the dog starts to gain some degree of self-control. At the same time the handler asserts himself or herself as pack leader. This will improve the dog's attention to the handler and, if corrections are well-timed, the dog's response to corrections.

One way to help the boisterous dog is to practice in a very quiet, indoor environment. Remove as many distractions as possible. Make sure the dog has eliminated and has had some exercise. Keep your movements smooth and confident. Don't talk to your excitable dog, and don't run or jump around. Calm, firm handling will communicate to your dog that you know what you are doing and that you are in charge. As you start to have success, increase distractions slowly. An excitable dog may always be excitable, but he can still be well trained. It is up to you to build his skills—slowly if necessary—and turn him into a great dog.

Chapter 26

Greeting People Without Jumping

DOGS WITH THIS SKILL are a pleasure to meet. They make a good first impression. Even people who do not like dogs too much can appreciate being in the presence of such self-control and good manners.

You probably have met dogs that are just the opposite. They bounce all over you, or they put their paws up on you, or they knock over your kids. They are not much fun.

If this describes *your* adopted dog, you need to do something about it. Not only will you, your family, your friends, and even strangers enjoy your dog a lot more, your dog will have the potential for a better life. Wouldn't it be better to have him calmly at your side when you open the front door for visitors? Wouldn't it be nice to be able to stop during a leash walk to greet someone and chat?

Wild-acting dogs don't get to do these things. They are banished to the garage or a back room whenever the doorbell rings. They get exercise in the backyard or not at all. They don't usually get to enjoy a sociable neighborhood walk, especially if they are big and strong. Keeping them under control whenever anyone approaches is just too exhausting.

Exiling a jumping dog to the backyard or the garage for many hours of the day can easily make the problem worse. After being socially isolated from visitors and their own families, many dogs get overly excited when they reconnect. This reinforces in the owner's mind that the dog cannot control himself and must be exiled. But exile gives the dog no opportunity to learn self-control. It is a vicious cycle of failure, with the dog the ultimate loser. A little obedience training would turn the whole situation around.

Teaching an old dog new tricks

Since your adopted dog is not a little puppy, he may have been jumping on people for months or even years. Can you really change this behavior? Absolutely. Follow the tale of Chester. It will help you understand how jumping gets started at a young age, how it turns into a habit, and what you can do about it. The specific training steps at the end of the chapter will take practice, but they will turn your jumper into a well-mannered dog that can go anywhere and meet anyone without losing control.

Case History: A Labrador Named Chester

When I met Chester, a chocolate Labrador retriever, a few years ago, he was eighteen months old. He was starting a new life in his *third* home.

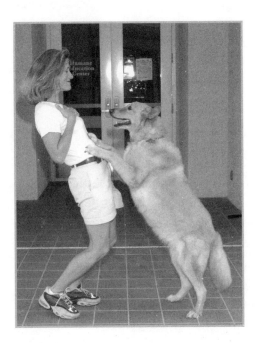

Thumper the Jumper is too big and strong to greet people like this. Fortunately, even an enthusiastic jumper can learn to greet people with all four feet on the ground.

Chester's first owners, the Westons, were a couple in their early seventies. Their children were grown, and they wanted a puppy. A Labrador breeder near where they lived told them to consider a smaller breed. The breeder felt that a Lab pup would be too much for them to handle, as Mrs. Weston was a petite woman with advanced arthritis in her hip. Her husband was frail and, because of long-term diabetes, had impaired vision. But they wanted a Labrador.

Puppies are not shoes

During a visit to the pet store in the local shopping mall, the Westons met Chester. He was eleven weeks old. According to what the salesperson at the store told them, he had just arrived from a breeder a day or two before.

When Mr. and Mrs. Weston first saw Chester in his cage in the pet store showroom, he was curled up sleeping. In the puppy greeting room he perked up somewhat but was still very calm and sweet. The couple interacted with Chester for fifteen minutes, fell in love, and purchased him.

When they reached their home, Chester was inquisitive about his new surroundings. He calmly poked around the house. Throughout most of the day he slept a lot. Aside from urinating once on the rug, Chester was a perfect puppy—for close to thirty-six hours. Then all hell broke loose.

Will the real Chester please stand up?

Chester suddenly had unlimited energy. He would race circles around his owners. Any attempts to control him were fruitless. If the Westons grabbed hold of him, Chester would wiggle and bite. In fact, Chester made them both a little nervous.

As time went on, the situation got worse. Chester was growing like a weed, and the bigger he got, the bolder his behaviors became. His most bothersome behavior was jumping up on the Westons and anyone who visited them. He would jump on them for attention, often from behind and scratching the backs of their legs.

After a few months of being jumped on, Mr. Weston called the pet store for help. He was advised that he should put his knee up and knee Chester in the chest when he jumped on them. They were also told that if this did not work, to shake a soda can filled with pennies at him. Neither approach worked.

Chester only jumped more when the Westons attempted to knee him, and he would run around like a lunatic when the penny can was shaken at him. The end came one fateful morning when an unanticipated jump from Chester knocked Mrs. Weston to the ground. Fortunately she was not seriously injured, but this was the last straw.

About five months from the day the couple bought Chester from the pet store, they gave him away. He was eight months old. A neighbor across the street knew a nice man with a family that was looking for a dog.

Two wrongs never make a right

The St. Croix family consisted of a stay-at-home mom with two children and a dad who ran a busy dental practice. The children were four and two years old. A wild, out-of-control Labrador was hardly what they needed. But he joined their household anyway.

Chester kept barreling playfully into the four-year-old girl, and soon the child became frightened of him. Interestingly, Chester had the intuition not to be as rowdy around the toddler. Wisely, Mom was taking no chances and kept the two separated.

But Chester jumped all over Mrs. St. Croix every chance he got, scratching her legs and muddying her clothes. Before long she could not take being around him. To avoid having to deal with the dog, Mrs. St. Croix banished Chester to the laundry room for most of the day.

He actually behaved fairly well in the laundry room. Sometimes he whimpered and cried, but mostly he slept or chewed on a rawhide. But he became wild when Mr. St. Croix got home from work at night and let him out of the laundry room.

Mr. St. Croix tried to make the adoption work. He enrolled Chester in a Saturday-morning dog obedience class. Unfortunately, he and Chester lasted only two weeks in the class. There were eighteen dogs

Common Mistakes That Encourage Jumping

If your adopted dog is bouncier than a tennis ball, the training exercises in this chapter are essential. But don't undo all your hard work by unintentionally encouraging your dog's jumping behavior. Consider these common mistakes. Correct as many as you can to help your jumper learn to keep his feet on the ground.

* Leaping for treats or a toy. Although this can be a fun trick, it encourages jumping. It also strengthens the dog's leg muscles for stronger jumping and risks injury to his hips and legs if he slips or lands roughly.

* Picking up your little dog to say hello, snuggling him around your face. This is normally a fine way to greet a dog. But if he's a jumper, lifting him up can encourage jumping. Better to make him sit and then bend down to say hello.

* Allowing your big dog to put his feet up on your hip or shoulders. This, too, contradicts your training efforts of teaching him to greet people with all four feet on the ground.

* Constantly being unprepared at the front door, without a leash and collar. You should put these on your dog every time someone knocks so that you can practice appropriate greeting skills. Consistency is the key to undoing a jumping habit. Training efforts are wasted if the dog frequently gets out of your control and is allowed to jump.

in the class, and the owners spent the majority of class time walking around in circles saying "Heel." Chester pulled on the leash and ignored Mr. St. Croix's commands.

Besides, it was Chester's nonstop jumping that was the big problem. The trainer's suggestion to stop Chester's jumping behavior was the knee-in-the-chest method. Mr. St. Croix had been trying this at home to no avail. He told the obedience instructor that kneeing Chester only seemed to get him wild and make him jump more.

The obedience instructor suggested that Mr. St. Croix grab Chester's two front paws when he jumped up and then pinch between his toes. When Chester's front feet were back on the ground, Mr. St. Croix was to praise him. This technique proved to be very awkward. He had a hard time even getting hold of Chester's feet, and when he did the dog tried to bite him. Mr. St. Croix knew that his wife could never do this procedure.

Finally Mr. St. Croix had to admit that he, too, was tired of being jumped on when he came home every night. He did not want to listen to his family complain about the dog every day. After several failed attempts to find a new home for Chester, he dropped him off at the county shelter. Chester stayed at the shelter for three weeks before he was once again adopted.

Happily ever after

Fortunately for Chester, he came to the attention of the Adopt-a-Dog organization based in Greenwich, Connecticut. This organization's function is to screen dogs in the pounds and shelters of the greater New York area and to find homes for them. The organization not only has a high success rate of placing dogs in homes, it also is successful in finding homes where the dog appropriately fits in and ends up staying. A big reason for this success is an experienced staff. They have the ability to expertly screen dogs and owners to be sure that they will be compatible together.

Finding a dog and owner who are a good match for each other is not always possible. But it was in Chester's case. The Smothers family could not have been more appropriate. The parents were in their late thirties with a twelve-year-old son. While the boy was in school during the week, Mom and Dad worked out of offices in their home. Family weekends were spent hiking and camping. Winter activities included cross-country skiing. A big, active Labrador would be a perfect companion.

Training days

The first day that I met Chester I was once again flabbergasted that such a great dog had been given away. Don't get me wrong. It was very apparent that his behavior needed some shaping up. He greeted me, of course, by jumping.

Right from the beginning, I communicated that jumping was unacceptable. I growled "Nhaa!" and then bent over and made him sit. I did so by sliding my right hand through his collar and then pushing down on his backside with my other hand.

When I took hold of his collar, Chester mouthed my arm. Again, I growled "Nhaa!" and he immediately stopped. It never ceases to amaze me how well a little canine communication works!

"Jumping on us and anyone that he meets is Chester's biggest problem," explained Mr. Smothers. "Other than that he is a pretty good dog."

Why dogs jump

I explained to the family that there are two reasons that dogs jump up on people. One reason is that they are seeking acknowledgment and attention. The other is to assert dominance.

Chester may have been motivated by both goals when he jumped on me as I entered the Smotherses' house. He was obviously excited to have a new visitor in the house, and he wanted attention. But jumping was also a way to see if I was someone that he could push around.

I explained to his owners that by using specific obedience techniques we would teach Chester to view them as pack leaders. Our goal also was to condition Chester to sit in order to gain what he wanted: attention and acknowledgment from people that he greeted.

In order to achieve this goal, Chester had to master three basic obedience skills. One was to sit immediately on command. Another was to stay sitting until released. The third was to stop doing whatever he was doing immediately when the Smotherses growled "Nhaa!"

These goals could not be met during one obedience lesson. However, I could teach the Smothers family the skills needed to teach these things to Chester. To be successful they had to practice every day until new habits were formed. Remember, dogs form habits by consistently repeating behaviors. If you want your dog to sit whenever he greets you, your family members, or other acquaintances, you have to teach him to do so and practice until it's a habit.

I'm happy to report that Chester (and his owners) learned this lesson well. I bumped into the Smothers family about a year later as they stood on a sidewalk talking to some friends. Chester was clipped to his leash and sat calmly at Mr. Smothers's side. I went over to say hello. Chester stood up, wiggling his body and wagging his tail with excitement—but his four feet never left the ground.

"Sit," I told him. And sure enough, Chester sat. I rubbed his chest and ears, greeting him warmly. Bravo, I thought to myself—obedience training once again saves the day, and the dog.

Step One: Bend Over and Make Him Sit, Every Time

Whether you are handling a new puppy or an adolescent or adult dog, you must make the effort to bend over and compel the dog to sit

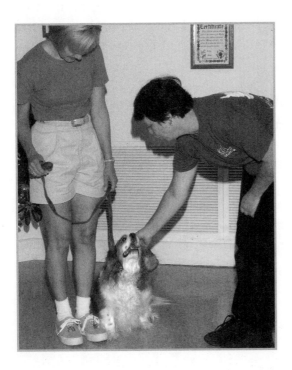

Simulated greetings help a dog to overcome jumping behavior. While the handler supervises a Sit-Stay, a helper says hello. Practice this frequently, with doorbells, knocks at the door, and walks into town to reinforce good greeting behavior.

whenever he greets you. Don't worry about his ability to greet others at this point. Starting today, do just what I did in the description above. Anticipate your dog's jumping and get your hands on his collar and on his rump. Place him into a sit, and then calmly say hello. Too much enthusiasm on your part may get him too hyped up and make him more difficult to handle.

If your dog is big and strong, this may not be easy. Some owners scoot their energetic dogs out into the yard as soon as they come home so the dog can run around for a minute or two. Then they can do a controlled greeting. Others clip a training collar and leash on the dog right away to get the leverage of an extra handling tool. Others grab the dog's collar as they open the kennel crate door, holding on to the dog before he has a chance to overpower them.

Step Two: Simulated Greetings

Once you reach a point in training where your dog will sit on command, stay until released, and respond properly to "Nhaa!" you can begin to practice simulated greetings. However, there is no need to wait until your dog is perfect with these basic skills. As long as he has some level of competence, you can get started. However, if it is a struggle to make him sit or he can only stay sitting for a few seconds, he's not ready. Practice a little longer on the basics.

This exercise allows the dog to practice greeting people many times in a simulated setting. For training purposes, these practice greetings are very contrived. When your dog becomes proficient with this procedure, you will begin to make the greeting circumstances more realistic.

The goal of this exercise is to teach your dog to accept being greeted and petted by different people without jumping up or reacting adversely. The more proficient he is at sit-stay, the more effective this procedure will be. To practice this exercise you will need a helper.

* Start with your dog sitting at your left side.
* Tell him, "Stay." Watch him closely. Remember you are doing the Sit-Stay exercise.

* Have a friend or family member knock on your door or ring the doorbell.
* Using a clear voice, say, "Come in." Be sure to keep your dog in a Sit-Stay at your left side when the greeter enters your house.
* Exchange verbal greetings with the helper.
* If your dog attempts to move, growl "Nhaa!" Use the leash to keep your dog sitting at your side. Do not restrain your dog with a tight leash. Give a gentle jerk and release to keep him sitting.
* Have the greeter approach your dog. If your dog remains sitting, have the greeter say hello to your dog by using his name and saying a few words to him in a pleasant, soothing manner.
* Remember that your main job is to keep your dog sitting and staying. As the helper approaches your dog, it is okay for both you and the greeter to say "Stay," if you feel it will help.
* If the dog remains sitting, have the greeter let your dog sniff the back of his or her hand. After doing this, have your helper briefly pet your dog's head. If your dog does not remain sitting at your side, have the examiner back off as you correct the dog with a growl— "Nhaa!"—and a jerk and release on the training collar. Your dog only gets attention from the visitor if he remains in a Sit-Stay.
* If your dog accepts the attention and remains in a Sit-Stay at your side, praise him warmly.

Repeat this procedure six times or more each session. Fortunately, dogs are pack animals and have a built-in greeting ritual. This means that every time your helper comes through the door, your dog is going to expect to be greeted. This allows you to repeat this exercise many times each training session. The repetition will develop in your dog a pattern of behavior and eventually a habit of a mannerly greeting.

If your dog is an energetic type and is easily stimulated, the greeter can start by simply saying hello to your dog. As this exercise becomes more familiar to your dog, the greeter can give him a quick pat on the head or a scratch on the chest.

Your job as the handler is to keep your dog in a Sit-Stay at your left side no matter what happens. Your dog's job is to stay and accept being greeted while sitting. The greeter's job is to interact with your dog *only* when he is sitting and under control.

Step Three: Make It More Natural

When your dog will sit and stay calmly when he is approached and petted by several different friends and family members, you can begin to make the greeting process more realistic.

After the greeter knocks or rings the doorbell, have your dog stay while you go and open the door and let the person in. Watch your dog as you head for the door. If your dog breaks the stay, say "Nhaa!" using a guttural tone. Be sure that your vocal correction is delivered as your dog is starting to get up. After the fact is too late.

After your vocal correction, calmly approach your dog and get hold of his leash. Bring him back to the spot from where he broke the stay. Replace him in a sitting position, and repeat the Stay command. Ask your helper to go back outside and try it again.

If your dog continually breaks the stay when you walk away from him, it means that he is not ready for this advanced step. Go back to practicing Step Two. With repetition he will get better.

Step Four: In the Real World

When your dog becomes proficient with greeting people while sitting and staying, employ this technique on the street. Whenever you meet people while out for a walk, make your dog sit. Say "Stay," and have your acquaintance greet your dog. If he gets rowdy when your friend speaks to or attempts to pet him, correct him with a "Nhaa!" and replace him in a Sit-Stay. Try it again. Remember, practice makes perfect.

Another Case Study: Crea, the Worst Jumping Dog I Ever Owned

Crea, my springer spaniel, proved why there is a "spring" in springer. She was a terrible jumper. She loved people and went wild whenever she was greeted. Of all the dogs that I have owned over the years, one of my biggest training challenges was to teach Crea not to jump on people.

From the day I brought her home as a small puppy, I started bending over and sitting her every time I greeted her. When she mastered the Sit-Stay exercise, we regularly practiced simulated visits at the front door.

During the first several years of Crea's life we lived on Nantucket Island. In the summer the downtown streets are filled with people, providing a great setting to practice greeting skills. Hardly anybody could resist saying hello to and petting a cute little springer pup. I had literally dozens of opportunities to practice greeting people without jumping.

Using the techniques described in this chapter has made Crea tremendously better, but truthfully, she is not perfect. Because of her breed and personality, she is easily stimulated. There are times when I still put her on the leash to make her sit and stay when guests are arriving. Although she is not perfect and probably never will be, she is vastly improved. Without this training, she would have been a real nuisance to live with.

What happens after you say hello?

Owners often ask me this question about this exercise: "Even if my dog greets my guest from a Sit-Stay, won't he just jump all over the person as soon as I release him from the stay?"

The answer is, probably not. Remember that the whole jumping thing is motivated by our dogs' need to be greeted and acknowledged whenever they meet people. When that need has been fulfilled, most dogs are not motivated to jump on people, unless it is to dominate them.

These dominant dogs, plus those that may still want to bug your guests for continued attention, need a second training step to manage the situation. The dog needs to be placed in a Down-Stay. A dog cannot jump on anyone while he is lying down and staying. Down-Stay is an indispensable control exercise for all sorts of situations, including these. Chapter 23 describes how to teach it to your dog.

A Third Case Study: Using Techniques Properly

I had a client on Nantucket who owned a very rambunctious collie mix. This dog was around eleven months old. She jumped on everyone! She did well with the training lessons despite living in a chaotic household. Her owners did the best that they could, between tennis and sailing, to find time to work with her. But before they had completed my entire training course, the summer was almost over and they were headed back to New York State.

Fortunately I had some engagements off-island in the next month and would not be far from their town. We made arrangements to complete the training course in New York.

On the scheduled evening of our next meeting, I showed up at their front door. After I rang the doorbell, I heard the mom's voice from inside the house call out to one of the children, "Don't open the door yet."

I assumed that Mom was getting set up and that when the door opened, the collie would be in a Sit-Stay at her side, waiting to be greeted without jumping.

But that was not what happened. When the door opened, Mom had her hand through the collar of a lunging collie and was shouting, "This procedure doesn't work!"

My response was, "It sure doesn't work the way you do it. Where is your leash? Make him sit at your side. Tell him to stay."

The moral of this story is that when all else fails, follow the instructor's advice. Training techniques only work well if you carry them out correctly.

Methods You Should Avoid

You have probably heard about one or more of these "training methods" to control jumping. They are all terrible. Here's why.

Kneeing the dog in the chest

The theory behind the popular "kneeing method" is that a knee in the chest is disagreeable, and dogs learn to avoid disagreeable experiences.

The flaw in the theory is that too many dogs interpret the knee in the chest as attention. Granted, it is negative attention, but it's attention nevertheless. If attention is what your dog wants, negative attention is better than no attention. As a result, your dog will continue the jumping behavior.

Increasing the force of the knee in the chest to make the experience more disagreeable is risky. A close veterinarian friend of mine, Chuck Noonan of Weston, Connecticut, has seen several cases where owners kneed their dogs too violently and caused injury. He showed me the X-rays of their broken or fractured bones. I advise that you do *not* knee your dog.

Ignoring the jumping behavior

A method that is currently in vogue with certain trainers is to simply ignore the dog when he jumps on you (or does any other unwanted behavior, for that matter). These trainers, who seem to avoid ever correcting dogs for fear of hurting their feelings, suggest that you turn your back on the dog, be quiet, and say nothing.

The theory here is that your dog is looking for attention and when he finally tires of mauling you, he will sit. When he does so, you are to reward him, and in time, he will figure out to sit instead of jump up when he wants your attention.

The good news about the turn-your-back method is that you certainly are not going to risk injuring your dog. But the bad news is that your dog is going to risk injuring you! With most dogs, this is an ineffective training technique.

Perhaps if the dog did stop jumping and eventually sat—and was quickly rewarded—he just might figure out that the way to gain attention was to sit. Unfortunately, most dogs will not react this way. In fact, it is more plausible that the dog will continue to jump on his owner's chest, back, or sides.

To make matters worse, many dogs will interpret the owner's turning away as a submissive posture and take advantage of it. The dog will continue to jump and perhaps even nip the owner. A handler's willingness to accept these "attacks" sends a message to the dog that the handler is subordinate. That's a great way to undermine a pack-leader image and bring failure to obedience training efforts.

And realistically, I think it is impossible to be quiet and say nothing when a seventy-five-pound dog is jumping on you and scratching your legs! There doesn't seem to be any common sense in this method. Almost *never* will ignoring a dog's behavior affect that behavior and change it for the better.

Grabbing the dog's feet and pinching between the toes

The theory behind this method is that when the dog jumps up and the owner pinches his feet, it will hurt. When the owner releases the dog's feet and they are back on the ground, the owner will praise the dog. The dog will choose what is agreeable and avoid what is disagreeable. Sound good? Here are the facts.

This method is both impractical and foolish. I have been training dogs for thirty years, and I do not have the speed, reflexes, and coordination to grab the front feet of most dogs, especially when they are jumping up. Now how is the typical dog owner going to do this? Can you immediately get your hands on a bouncing little Jack Russell terrier? Are you going to tell your eight-year-old child to pinch the Rottweiler between the toes?

Actually that is not the foolish aspect of the technique; it's the impractical part. The foolish part is purposely hurting your dog's feet for any reason. Dogs are extremely sensitive and protective of their feet. It is important that your dog learn to trust you to handle his feet. You, your veterinarian, and your dog groomer are all going to need to be able to handle your dog's feet throughout his life. If you grab his feet and pinch between his toes, you will very quickly undermine your dog's trust and create a major handling problem.

Even *if* you were able to gracefully grab your dog's feet and pinch his toes, and even *if* you were not concerned about the backlash effects of hurting his feet, this is still an inferior method. It does not teach the dog a better, more appropriate way to greet people. All you would end up with is a dog that did not know how to appropriately greet someone. That's not training.

Part Five

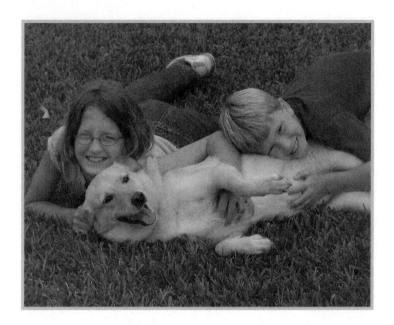

Additional Tips for Success

These chapters provide the final polish on a success-ful adoption. With guidance on exercise, grooming, and spaying and neutering—plus safe interactions with children and with other pets—you can be assured that your adopted dog will be a wonderful lifelong companion.

Chapter 27

Excercise Is a Must

ONE OF THE BEST WAYS to help strengthen your relationship with your newly adopted dog is to do things with him that involve physical activity. Regular exercise is just as important to a dog's physical and mental well-being as obedience training. In many cases, one cannot be achieved without the other.

My favorite motto that I use when I help new dog owners through puppyhood is "A tired puppy is a good puppy." This motto also applies to adolescent and adult dogs. Daily exercise provides all sorts of benefits to dogs. Consider this long list of advantages: Exercise strengthens muscle, reduces fat, eliminates stress, promotes a good appetite and regular elimination, fights boredom, helps with socialization, and inspires sleep.

Dogs that receive regular exercise are dramatically less prone to behavioral problems around the house. Add some obedience training and careful supervision, and you have the ingredients for turning out one terrific dog.

Physical fun with your dog is limited only by commonsense safety issues and your own imagination. Consider this story: During a beach hike last year with my springer spaniel, Crea, I met a middle-aged man paddling his two-person kayak in the shallow surf. I should call his vessel a two-*creature* kayak, as a black Lab was the other passenger, sitting calmly in front of him and enjoying the adventure. He told me they traveled by kayak (along the shoreline, not across deep water) to some remote beaches where they enjoyed hiking, swimming, and exploring together. Lucky dog.

I have met people who go on overnight backpacking adventures with their dogs. I have seen folks on rollerblades taking their dog for a run. Whenever our infant daughter went on a stroller walk with my wife, one of the dogs went along, too.

This chapter describes a variety of dog-appropriate exercise and fun activities. But don't be limited by these suggestions. Share your life and your interests with your adopted dog. That's what he's there for.

Dog Hikes

Dogs love to go for hikes in the woods, through fields, or along beaches. I'm convinced that they view such adventures as hunting. They can move around freely, investigating interesting scents, listening

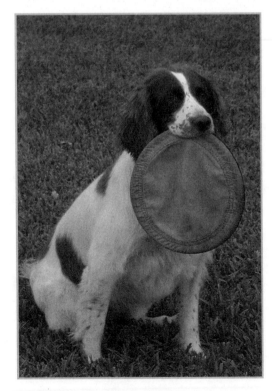

My energetic spaniel, Crea, would have been a nightmare pet without frequent exercise. She likes to chase a soft disk and will bring it back to me over and over again. When Crea was young, I always got tired long before she did.

to birds and other wildlife, watching people and other dogs. Best of all, they are hunting with *you*. It is a great way to reinforce to your adopted dog that you and he now belong in the same pack. By directing the speed and direction of the hike, you also reinforce your role as the pack's leader. This will greatly help with your obedience training efforts and with controlling your dog's behavior in general.

Hiking does not have to mean rugged terrain, lug-soled boots, a knapsack of supplies, and a map and compass. A long, off-leash stroll down your favorite beach can be a dog hike. A walk through a pretty field of wildflowers can be a dog hike. So can a two-mile jog along a dirt road.

Ideally, a dog would like to go out adventuring every day. But most of us cannot plan our schedules around dog hikes. Try for a thirty-minute or one-hour dog hike several times a week. It will be great exercise, and it will leave you with a dog that is both mentally and physically content.

Consider this

Dog hikes are out of the question if your adopted dog is going to run off and not come when called. Stick with leash walks for now. After you have completed obedience training, you may be able to hike with your dog. Be sure to reinforce your dog's Come on Command training from time to time. Dogs can get rusty with this important exercise, but off-leash freedom absolutely requires that a dog respond to your call.

Dogs are allowed to run off-leash in all sorts of places. Do respect leash laws, however. Check for signs posted at park entrances, beach access points, or other public areas. Ask landowners if it is okay to hike in their fields. The farther you are from densely populated areas, the more choices you will probably have for off-leash fun. But even big cities have dog parks. Many are fenced so dogs can run around safely.

Be sure that your dog is friendly with people and dogs that you may encounter along the trail. It would be irresponsible—and possibly criminal—to unclip Cujo's leash, knowing that he is aggressive and dangerous around others. A dog like that must be exercised in other ways.

Leash Walks

A very wise veterinarian that I knew used to tell his clients who owned hyper dogs, "You can walk him to China and never tire him out. He needs to run!"

He may have been right, but, fortunately, not all dogs are hyper. Walking can provide plenty of exercise for many dogs. A 30-to-60-minute leash walk is not only good for dogs, it's great for humans. If you live in the city or are not capable of hiking with your dog, go for a walk. Go every day if possible. It will be good for both of you.

Consider this

If your dog thinks that you are a sled and he is a sled dog, you need to make some changes. Being dragged down the street on the end of the leash is no fun, and it can harm your dog's throat.

If this describes your dog, you need to teach him the Controlled Walking exercise found in Chapter 25. You will be amazed at how much difference it makes. Once Controlled Walking has been mastered, dog walks will be fun. You can take your baby along in the stroller, or you can window-shop or run errands in town.

Leash walks also provide great opportunities for mini-obedience practice. Your dog can sit and stay at your side while you wait at a corner for traffic to clear. He can greet people without jumping when you see a neighbor and stop to say hello. He can lie down and stay if you want to sit on a park bench and read the newspaper. Use these opportunities to reinforce your dog's skills and to stimulate his mind. Pet-oriented obedience skills are for everyday life. Put them to use!

A word of caution: If you are an athletic person who runs, jogs, or "power walks" great distances, you should not assume that your dog can do the same. Certainly some dogs are trained athletes, with the strength and endurance for long runs. But most any dog that you adopt will not come to you ready for such a strenuous workout. Speak to your veterinarian about your dog's physical condition before you start exercising vigorously together. Consider the dog's age, physical soundness (especially his hips and legs), breathing impairments (such as found in bulldogs, Boston terriers, and pugs), and coat. Consider also the surface you will be running or walking on and the temperature and humidity during your workout. Inflicting tendinitis, abraded foot pads, and heat stroke on your dog is abuse, not exercise.

Retrieving

Some dogs love to play fetch. Retrievers may have been bred to bring back ducks, but tennis balls are just about as good. Many terriers, spaniels, shepherds, and all sorts of other dogs think so, too. If your adopted dog is tennis-ball-crazy or Frisbee-obsessed, put this to good use as a way to exercise him. Twenty to thirty minutes of retrieving fun will poop most dogs out. And you barely have to move!

Consider this

Not all dogs like to retrieve. If your dog has no interest in retrieving, fetching games will not work for you. Others dogs do like to run after objects and grab them; they just don't like to bring them back. Some dogs bring them back but won't give them up.

If your dog enthusiastically fetches a ball or Frisbee but then plays "catch me if you can," try this. Have two tennis balls or Frisbees. After your dog runs out and grabs the thrown ball, get his attention by calling him. Then show him the other ball. Once he zeros in on the ball in your hand, encourage him to come to you.

Chances are good that when he reaches you, he will drop the first ball because he will want the other one. As he drops the first ball, say, "Drop." (My dogs all learned to drop a ball—or just about anything—on command by practicing this way.) Praise your dog enthusiastically when he drops the ball and then throw the second one. This rotation technique helps many dogs overcome their possessiveness of the object and teaches them how to actually play fetch. Even these training sessions will help tire out your dog.

When your dog gets good with the fetch game and drops the object on command, you can get your kids in on the fun. My springer spaniel, Crea, would play nonstop in the backyard with anyone of any age who tossed the ball. Even when my daughter was a preschooler, she could send a tennis ball down our grassy hill, and Crea would fetch it and drop it at her feet for another toss. As long as your adopted dog does not get too wild during play, your kids can exercise him and enjoy some fresh air and fun, too.

Swimming

Swimming is a great form of exercise for a dog. It is particularly good for dogs with arthritic problems in their hips and shoulder joints. This is because the impact on joints during swimming is far less than when running or jogging. If you do have an arthritic dog, discuss his capabilities with your veterinarian. You should not overdo any physical activity, even swimming.

Icy-cold water should be avoided, particularly with dogs with joint problems. Ocean surf and riptides can be dangerous. So can fast-moving rivers and streams. Avoid rough water, no matter how strong a swimmer you have. And if you live in Florida or some other warm region, watch out for gators!

Consider this

Almost all dogs can swim and will enjoy doing so if they are properly introduced to water. Never throw or drag a dog into water. Slow and steady exposure to gentle bodies of water will teach your dog to feel confident and to love water.

Unfortunately, many adopted dogs were previously owned by less conscientious owners. If your dog was improperly introduced to water, he may have learned to fear and hate it. Be patient with him and do not expect too much too soon. Reintroduction to water may be very difficult if your adopted dog is over a year old. Be prepared for the possibility that he may never be a swimmer.

And a word of caution to all owners: Use extreme caution if you choose to swim with your dog. Dogs may tire out or panic or simply want to get close to you. The results can be disastrous if the dog tries to climb on you, pushing you under. For safety's sake, stay clear of your dog while swimming in any water that is over your head.

Doggie Ping-Pong

This game requires two people and is best played on a beach or in a big yard or field. It is a great way to tire your dog out. Even better, it reinforces the Come and Sit commands as you play.

Start with your dog sitting near you. Have your helper stand fifty to seventy feet away. Using a clear and pleasant voice, have your helper call your dog's name followed by the command "Come!" As usual, the person calling the dog should encourage him after giving the command. Clap hands, for example, and say "Good dog!" in an enthusiastic tone.

As the dog comes racing forward, the helper should show your dog an object of attraction. A ball or squeaky toy usually works well—anything that gets the dog's attention. When the dog arrives, the helper should sit the dog and reward him with a piece of doggie biscuit.

After about twenty seconds or so, call your dog back to you. When he reaches you, make him sit and food reward him. Wait twenty seconds and then have your helper call the dog again.

Repeat this technique of calling the dog back and forth between you and your helper a dozen times or so. Be sure to really verbally encourage the dog after calling his name and giving the command "Come!" The goal is to get him running as fast as possible as he enthusiastically responds to each command. This game really tires dogs out, and it's constructive at the same time.

Consider this

This game does require two people. If you cannot find someone to help, this one is not for you.

If there is a chance that your dog may not come when called and will take off instead, try this game in a fenced area. You can also allow the dog to drag a thirty-foot long line when you play. If he does not come, go to the end of the long line and step on it. Do not reel the dog in like a fish on a line.

After you have stepped on the long line, pick it up and run away from your dog. Running away will cause him to chase you. When he does come running, squat down and entice him to you with a piece of doggie biscuit. Praise him warmly when he comes to you, and give him a piece of the biscuit.

If the dog comes well but does not sit on command, each handler may have to hold a leash when playing Doggie Ping-Pong. Clip the leash to the dog's collar when he reaches you. Give the food reward and then make him sit and stay for about twenty seconds. Unclip the leash when the other handler is ready to call him.

Find It!

This is a great game that many dogs really have fun playing. It stimulates their brain and tires them out at the same time. It is perfect for a rainy day or a cold winter night, because you play it indoors (although playing outside would work, too).

Dogs need a few skills to play this game. First, they must have a good sense of smell. I have never met a dog that did not! Second, they must enjoy fetching. They also must be able to lie down and stay reliably.

To start, place your dog in a down position and tell him, "Stay." Show him a tennis ball, squeaky toy, or anything that he loves.

While he is lying down and watching you, hide the ball somewhere in the area where you are playing. A family room works great. Part of your job is to avoid hiding the ball immediately. Walk around the room, pretending to place the ball in various spots, such as on a chair, under a table, next to the sofa, etc. Touch the ball in each of these locations (five or six are plenty). At some point, actually leave the ball in one of the hiding spots. Then continue on, acting as though you are still putting the ball in different places.

When you are finished, return to your dog. Wait about ten seconds and then release your dog from the stay. Give the command "Find it!"

The objective of the game is for your dog to search the room methodically and to find the ball. Most dogs that I have played with will check every spot that I touched as I was hiding the ball. In fact, they usually start at the first place they saw me go. If they are not immediately successful finding the ball, the nose starts working. Good! Eventually they almost always sniff out the ball.

When the dog does succeed in finding the ball, praise him exuberantly. As you praise, allow him to carry the ball in his mouth for a minute or two before you take it to play again. Strutting around with the "prey" in his mouth while the pack leader lavishes praise is very fulfilling to a dog. Crea wiggles and wags all over while I tell her what a smart, clever girl she is. It is so much fun to watch her "hunt" and find it that we often play ten or twenty rounds before ending.

Dogs can get really good at this game. To make it more challenging, you can have your dog wait out of sight while you hide the ball. Then he really has to use his nose, right from the beginning. Or you can expand the play area to include several rooms. Friends of mine play this game in the dark! Their spaniel hunts for the ball completely by scent and comes up with it every time.

Consider this

This is a game that dogs improve at the more they play. At first it may be necessary to help your dog. Walk around the room with him, encouraging him with the command "Find it." Point to the different areas where you made believe that you hid the ball. Then direct him to the correct hiding spot. Help him be successful, and also give lots of praise when he is.

I have one friend who played this game using her two young daughters as the "objects" to find. The girls would hide in the house and, eventually, in a wooded field behind their house. On command ("Find the girls!") their dog would search for them until the girls were found. This was a fun game for everyone, and it developed a canine skill that could come in handy if the girls were truly lost.

Case Study: The Energetic Irish Setter

Several decades ago the Irish setter was an extremely popular breed in the United States. In the 1970s I met two Irish setters that were owned by a friend of a friend. After just a few hours hiking in the woods and playing with these two exuberant dogs, I decided that I wanted an Irish setter. I was smitten by the breed's beauty. So was the rest of the country.

Throughout much of the 1970s the Irish setter was the number one breed registered by the American Kennel Club. Unfortunately, these dogs also ended up in shelters in record numbers. This is because they were so highly energetic. The average family could not live compatibly with them.

Carrousel's Jason, utility dog

Jason was not a shelter dog that I rescued. I bought Jason as a puppy from a dog breeder in 1972. He was the first dog that I owned on my own. At the time I knew nothing about dogs or dog training. My objective as a dog owner was simply to have a companion to love and to take hiking in the woods.

A calm Irish setter?

Only a few months after I got Jason I changed jobs, and overnight my life had completely changed. I became a veterinarian's assistant. One of the comments my new employer made when he met my six-month-old pup was, "Boy, this is the only calm Irish setter that I have ever met."

"Oh, he's not calm," I replied. "He's tired." That's because exercise was a big part of Jason's life.

Over time I realized that many people failed in their attempts to train their Irish setters because their dogs were so mentally wound up. In that mental state, dogs are not under emotional control. When dogs are out of emotional control, they cannot learn. Daily hikes with Jason put him in a mentally receptive place that allowed him to learn and, in turn, to be well-behaved.

I am still proud of the fact that Jason was the very first Irish setter from Connecticut to earn a Utility Dog obedience title through the American Kennel Club. The Utility Dog title requires much more than basic obedience skills. At the time, it was the highest level of achievement in obedience competition. A lot of people were surprised that any Irish setter could be so well trained.

Jason was not only a successful obedience trial competitor, he was also a great canine citizen and a loving friend. I always attributed my success with Jason to adequate exercise. I guarantee that exercise will help your dog, too.

Chapter 28

Grooming Tips

THIS IS A GREAT PLACE to put your dog's obedience skills to use. Dogs that come on command can easily be rounded up at bath time. Dogs that can stay in place are a pleasure to bathe and dry. They easily can be brushed out and combed. Without a struggle these dogs can have well-trimmed nails, clean ears, and polished teeth. And while you do these things with your dog, your back won't go out and your good humor will stay intact. This is one of many, many situations where an obedient dog is a real joy.

My wife and writing partner, Barbara McKinney, is the dog bather in our house. She has been successful at helping all of our dogs over the years to enjoy—or at least to calmly accept—a bath. Here is her advice.

A Trip to the Groomer

Depending on your dog's breed, your personal preferences, and your budget, a professional groomer may be a regular part of your dog's life. Every few weeks some dogs go to the groomer's shop for a thorough once-over: bath, fur clipping, ears, nails, etc. If this will be part of your routine with your adopted dog, here are a few tips for making (and keeping) it a positive experience for everyone.

Choose a groomer based on his or her professional reputation, not on the size advertisement in the phone book or the extreme convenience to your home. Ask your veterinarian and dog-owning neighbors who they use. The groomer you select should be known for treating dogs kindly. He or she should have high standards of safety and hygiene. Ideally, the dog should spend only enough time there for the grooming process. If all day is necessary, bathroom breaks and fresh water are a must.

A good professional groomer has enough dog handling experience to help almost any dog enjoy (or at least tolerate) a bath. If you have any doubts about your adopted dog's ability to accept being groomed, discuss this with the groomer before your first appointment. He or she may want to meet your dog first.

Be sure to share any background information about your adopted dog that may affect the groomer's work. A dog that was beaten with a hairbrush (yes, I knew one) may panic or become aggressive when it's time to be brushed. Help your groomer—and your dog—be successful by sharing these kinds of details if you know them.

Some dogs may not adjust well to the multi-dog setting of a busy grooming shop. It can get a little noisy. Barking, blow dryers, ringing telephones, and perhaps a radio playing can all add up. Actually, this may seem normal to dogs that once lived in an animal shelter! But other dogs may find it extremely unnerving. If your adopted dog is one of them, consider finding an alternative. Perhaps your groomer would give you an after-hours appointment. Some groomers work out of specially equipped vans and drive up to your door for personalized, on-site dog grooming services. Or you could do it yourself.

Doing It Yourself

Here are some tips for a basic, at-home grooming. For the finer points of dog grooming, consult a professional. John once tried to give his adopted poodle, Jossie, a clipping. Big mistake. She handled it just fine, because he was gentle and careful with her. But the work took forever, and the result looked pretty bad. Poodle fur requires a lot more expertise than he had.

For the rest of our dogs (mostly all short-haired), a bath and towel-dry were easy. If you have never bathed a dog, or suspect that your adopted dog has never had a bath, consider these suggestions. With a little effort, your dog will not only behave well, he will smell, look, and feel great, too.

Tub time

Safety first. Put a nonslip mat on the bottom of the tub or sink where you will bathe your dog. A slippery, wet surface can easily make your dog panic and want to jump out, or he could slip and fall, causing injury to himself or to you.

Round up everything you will need before the bath starts. Get the shampoo, a spray hose or pitcher for rinsing, a stack of old towels, and anything else you can think of. You don't want to leave a wet or soapy dog alone while you run around looking for supplies. He probably won't be there when you get back, or he will have shaken off several times, flinging water and suds everywhere. (I've learned this the hard way!)

If you are able, lift your dog into the tub or sink rather than getting him to jump in. You will minimize the risk that he might slip and fall, and you avoid showing him than he can get into the tub or sink at any time, which is not something I encourage with my dogs.

Use warm or tepid water for dog baths. I don't care how stoic your dog is, no warm-blooded creature likes to be soaked down with ice-cold water.

When your dog is in the tub, give the commands "Stand" and "Stay." Growl "Nhaa!" if he starts to move around. Your dog's job in the tub is to obey your commands. A dog that will stand and stay during a bath is an example of pet obedience training at its finest!

Always use dog shampoo to wash your dog, as human shampoo and other cleaning preparations (dish detergent, laundry soap, etc.) are not safe for a dog's skin and coat. Rinse well, and rinse again. Dry, itchy, or inflamed skin are often caused by shampoo residue.

I typically towel-dry my dogs and put them in a sunny, warm room to finish air-drying. If you need your dog dried more quickly, use a hand-held blow dryer. Keep it moving back and forth along the dog's coat to prevent burning his skin. Many dogs don't like the blow dryer's soft roar, however. In my opinion, it is not necessary to force it on a dog that fears it. Just use a big stack of towels to get him mostly dry.

To praise or not to praise?

A dog that is nervous during a bath needs to be handled properly so that he does not become more fearful. In fact, your goal should be getting him to relax and perhaps even enjoy the warm water, soapy massage, and soft towel-drying.

Our human instincts with a nervous person, especially a nervous child, are to calm their fears with soothing words. "It's okay, nothing bad is going to happen. Don't worry." This approach backfires with dogs. Dogs do not understand our exact words, but they do hear our voice tones, which sound like encouragement and praise. By verbally reassuring a nervous dog, you are actually reinforcing his nervous feelings.

It is best to say nothing. Be kind and firm with your handling, and if the dog tries to jump out or wiggle free, correct him with a growl— "Nhaa!" Then be quiet again. If and when you feel his body relax or his nervousness change to acceptance, turn on the praise. Keep it soft and soothing, however. Loud sounds in a tiled bathroom are usually amplified; they will unnerve anyone.

My yellow Lab, Bentley, was a bit nervous of new things, including baths. But he learned to accept them, even enjoying (as best as I could tell) the quiet praise and gentle massage associated with getting clean. My efforts to make his baths peaceful and pleasant paid off. Also, by giving him a job to do, such as Stand-Stay or Sit-Stay, I could help him focus on that obedience task and not worry quite so much about the bath.

How often to bathe?

Some dogs are groomed once a week. My Labs got bathed a few times a year. How often you bathe your own dog depends on many things, including personal preference. Does your dog sleep on your bed? Do you have a muddy backyard? Does his coat get mats or burrs? Is his fur long or short? Do you have a lot of light-colored rugs? These considerations will influence your bath schedule.

I do recommend that every dog be brushed or combed at least once a week, no matter how frequently he is bathed. By going over his coat regularly, you will get to know your dog's body and what looks and feels normal on him. You may find attached ticks that need removal, evidence of fleas that require eradication, cuts that need first-aid treatment, or small lumps that require veterinary care before they turn into big lumps. This weekly once-over is an important yet easy way to maintain your dog's health. A groomer or pet supply shop owner can guide you to the right kinds of brushes and combs for your dog's coat.

Although I have enjoyed the job of giving our family dogs their baths, John is the ears and nails expert in our house. Here's what he has to say on this important aspect of good grooming.

Ears and Nails

Clean ears and trimmed nails are essential to good grooming for any dog. Not only does this keep your dog looking and smelling good, it helps prevent ear infections, broken nails, and other problems.

I am always careful not to give out veterinary advice. If your dog has sore ears, excessive wax buildup, unusually long nails, a broken toenail, or any other problem that you do not feel confident handling, call your veterinarian. He or she can treat the problem and may show you how to handle it yourself in the future. The relatively small cost of an office visit and perhaps some medication are always preferable to the expense (for you) and the discomfort (for your dog) of letting a small ailment turn into a big, complicated mess.

Once a month is a good guideline for tending to most dogs' ears and nails. A gentle wipe inside the ear flap can whisk away any excess wax. Use a cotton ball or soft tissue wrapped around your finger. Do not use any special ear cleaner unless advised to do so by your veterinarian. Do not reach into the dog's ear canal. Any surface that you can easily see can be wiped clean. Your veterinarian should tend to excess wax or other problems deeper into the ear.

Trim your dog's nails only slightly. You risk cutting the blood vessel inside each nail if you cut back too far. Not only will that hurt your dog, it will make him less willing to allow you to trim his nails in the future. A little snip at the tip is usually sufficient. For unusually long or broken nails, see your vet.

As a general rule, dogs do not like having their nails trimmed, even when it is done carefully. Dogs are very protective of their feet. Yet they must allow you to handle their feet for cleaning, drying, nail trimming, and inspection for cuts or scrapes.

I have always had good success with teaching my dogs to accept nail trimming. Fortunately, I taught most of them this skill while they were puppies. You may have a harder time with a newly adopted adolescent or adult dog, especially if the dog has memories of painful clippings, rough handling, or other trauma related to his feet. Sadly, some dogs even need to be sedated by a veterinarian for this simple aspect of care.

If you regularly trim your dog's nails without a struggle, congratulations. Keep up the good work. If you need some pointers on how to

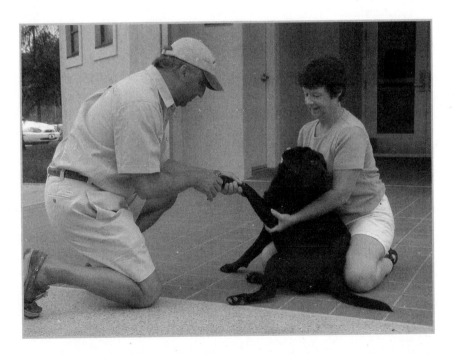

Nail clipping is an important part of good grooming. A helper can steady your dog and prevent him from pulling his paws away from you. Be sure to snip only the nail's tip. Otherwise the nails will bleed, and your dog will quickly learn to fear and hate nail clipping.

do it—or how to do it better—follow this training advice. With regular practice it may turn a difficult chore into a quick and easy process.

First, you must gain your dog's confidence when you handle his feet. A dog that is nervous and jumpy when his feet are touched certainly cannot hold still while you try for an accurate snip on each nail. Practice feet-handling! Sit on the floor with your dog several times each day and hold each paw in turn, gently touching each toe. When your dog accepts this, praise him in a soothing tone. If he enjoys doggie treats, give him one after you finish handling each foot.

If your dog struggles and pulls away when you touch his feet, tell him "Nhaa!" in a low, guttural tone. Then continue to handle his feet. Do the same thing if he growls or tries to mouth your hand. If your dog gets really nasty and tries to bite you, you will not be able to do the nail-clipping on your own. Get the help of a veterinarian or professional groomer.

Repeat this procedure several times a day for about two weeks. During this time, work on another procedure separately. Have your dog sit, show him the toenail clippers, and give him a doggie treat while you praise him. Touch the clippers to his feet, praising him and giving a doggie treat. If you are successful with these procedures after two weeks of practice, you can now try clipping his nails. You will need an assistant for this training.

Barbara is usually my assistant. She places the dog-in-training in a sitting position on her left side and kneels down next to him. She slides her right hand through the dog's collar. She reaches her left arm around the dog's back and uses her left hand to lift the dog's left front leg. She grasps around the dog's elbow, because it prevents the dog from pulling his leg back.

While she holds the leg, I sit in front of the dog, gently holding his foot and quickly snipping each nail. Then Barbara switches sides and we do the right foot.

To do the back feet, we have the dog lie down on his side. Sitting on the floor, Barbara holds him gently from behind and slightly lifts each hind leg while I clip the nails. After the procedure is complete, we both praise lavishly, and the dog gets a treat. Although most dogs are not thrilled about getting their nails done, they can learn to accept it without a fight.

And a reminder: The key to success is to avoid clipping too far. Just nick the tips of each nail to avoid cutting the blood vessel inside. Although your dog will not bleed to death if you do, cutting into this blood vessel (commonly called the "quick") will hurt your dog. And he will not want you to clip his nails again. If you do accidentally make your dog's toenail bleed, apply pressure with a paper towel for a few minutes to stop the bleeding. And try very hard not to make this mistake again. Struggle-free nail clipping depends on it.

Cleaning Teeth

No chapter on keeping your dog clean would be complete without mention of canine dental care. A generation ago—even just a decade ago—few people brushed their dog's teeth or even heard of doing it. That has changed. Veterinarians advise us to provide regular teeth brushing and periodic plaque scrapings if needed. Commercial pet foods advertise ingredients that are designed to promote dental health. And a survey of pet supply catalogs shows an interesting variety of doggie toothbrushes and toothpastes for that bright, healthy canine smile.

Your veterinarian is the best place to start for assessing the condition of your adopted dog's teeth. If thick buildups of plaque must be removed, your dog will be anesthetized in the vet's office so that it can be scraped off. My dogs have occasionally had this procedure, which is relatively simple but not inexpensive. A few times I have even used this opportunity to have small lumps removed or an X-ray taken.

Your veterinarian can recommend the best routine for at-home cleaning of your dog's teeth. Crunchy, dry kibble is said to be better for teeth than canned meat or moist food chunks. Teeth-healthy snacks include hard dog biscuits and crunchy produce, like carrots and apples.

With a little regular attention to your dog's teeth, ears, nails, and coat, you will have a clean pet and in all likelihood a healthy pet.

Chapter 29

Kids and Dogs: Play It Safe

"MOM, CAN WE get a dog? Pleeeease?"

It seems that dogs and kids go together like peanut butter and jelly. Look at Lassie and Timmy, Snoopy and Charlie Brown, Petey and the Little Rascals. (Boy, am I old!) Dogs and kids are well-known partners.

The vast majority of children love dogs and want to own one. If you grew up with a dog a few decades ago and have fond memories of that experience, you may want the same for your kids. I know I did.

Unfortunately, the realities of dog ownership and the dog–child relationship are not always the same as Hollywood portrays them to be. And our own memories of youthful dog ownership probably do not include the adult responsibilities that were involved, such as housebreaking, the cost of veterinary care, the time needed for training, the pressure to exercise and groom the dog, etc.

One of your jobs as a parent is to make responsible decisions for your family. If you want your children to enjoy the company of a family dog and to have lasting memories of a wonderful pet, this chapter will help. It includes safety guidelines plus tips for integrating the kids into your adopted dog's training and care.

What is the best kind of dog for my family?

I have received hundreds of phone calls over the years from families asking, "What would be the best kind of dog for my family?" When I ask who is in the family, a common response is "We have two children, a toddler, and a new baby on the way," or "We have a three-year-old and also a five-year-old in kindergarten."

A red flag goes up when I hear this. I have seen too many frustrated parents trying to juggle young kids and a dog, especially when the dog is a puppy or adolescent. I politely explain to these well-intentioned folks that there are a lot of challenges when adding a dog to a family with young children. (See Chapter 2, "What Are You Looking For?," for more on this topic.) I usually answer this question about the "best kind of dog" with my standard advice: "Do yourself a favor. Get a stuffed dog."

This is a glib answer, I admit. But I have seen too many adolescent

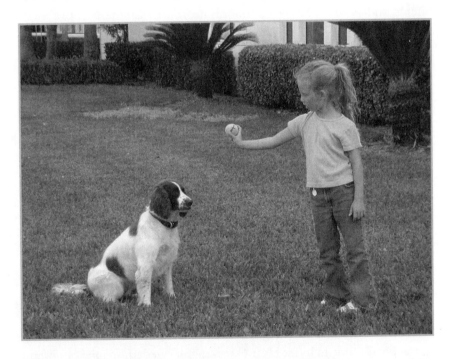

"Play" is what kids and dogs seem to do best. Supervision is important, especially when the kids are young and the adopted dog is new to your home.

dogs end up in pounds because families with young children often give up on the challenge of puppy-raising. It takes a lot of work to do it right!

However, I am careful not to underestimate the abilities of individuals. It is not my job to tell anyone that he or she is incapable of owning a dog. I have known a small number of families with young children who successfully raised puppies. I'm sure there were many days when they had second thoughts about it. Despite the challenges, they survived, and their puppies turned into nice, well-behaved adults. But statistically, they are the exception to the rule.

Small Children and Dogs

By nature, little kids are inconsistent beings. Nothing about a toddler or kindergarten kid says to a dog, "I'm in charge. You must follow direction from me." Their small size, high-pitched voices, erratic movements, and playful natures communicate, from a canine point of view, that small children are littermate youngsters, not dominant adults.

Puppies especially are inclined to bite and chew on kids in the same way that they would other puppies. They are testing their own dominance and the dominance or submissiveness of these youngsters. This usually leaves parents with screaming children and with puppies that end up in the proverbial dog house.

If you have adopted a puppy or an adolescent dog, this situation may sound familiar. You will need to tighten the ship and supervise, supervise, supervise. Come to your children's rescue if the dog gets too feisty. The dog must learn not to mouth *anyone* in the household, including the kids. Your corrective growl—"Nhaa!"—is needed every time.

Old Enough to Help

Until children are at least eight years old, their interactions with a dog are generally not helpful. Housebreaking, if needed, requires constant supervision. So does teaching a young dog to avoid chewing inappropriate household items. Parents who are busy supervising small children often cannot keep a close eye on dogs and kids simultaneously. The typical result is a pet that is ignored or exiled from the family.

After the age of eight, children can constructively help with the work that is required for canine care, as long as they have parental supervision. They can feed the pup and take him into the yard to eliminate. They can go with you on leash walks or go on their own if they are older. Kids love to play, and so do dogs. Also, children over eight

Think Through Your Adoption Plans

In my thirty years of experience with dogs and their families, I have found that the idea for getting a family dog is very often Dad's idea. Dad probably grew up with a dog, and he likes the idea that his kids will, too. Now that he has a house, a wife, a family, and a decent job, the only thing missing from this picture of domestic bliss is the family dog.

"A dog would be great for the kids," he tells his wife. She is more interested in caring for her two young children than in some dog, but she goes along with the idea. She likes dogs, too.

Unfortunately, Mr. Idealistic spends fifty-plus hours a week at the office. He's understandably tired in the evenings and likes to relax in front of the television. On weekends he cuts the grass or plays in a golf tournament or coaches the kids' tee-ball team—or all three. For the vast majority of time, he is unavailable for raising and training the family dog. That falls to his wife, who now has another family member to feed, supervise, exercise, and raise. It should come as no surprise that she does not have the time or the energy to do a very good job. I wouldn't either in her shoes.

If you are the dad reading this, think twice about what you are asking your spouse to do. Your young children come first, and they need a lot of attention. But so does a dog, if you want the dog to be a well-adjusted and well-behaved member of your family. If you are the mom reading this section, show it to your husband. And stand firm if you have doubts about the timing of this adoption. Doing it right is more important than doing it now.

years old can usually convince a dog that they are in charge, not the other way around.

Summer School for Kids and Dogs

In the late 1980s, Barbara and I offered a week-long program called Summer School for Kids and Dogs. The children ranged in age from eight to twelve years old. The dogs ranged in age from five months to five years old.

Every day for an hour the kid-and-dog teams showed up, and we taught them basic obedience exercises. It was a fun experience, because we love both dogs and children. Nevertheless, my grand conclusion at the end of the week was that *dogs do not listen well to children*. At least not nearly as well as they might listen to an adult.

Don't get me wrong—the kids had fun, and I think that they learned a lot. But it was evident that children were not viewed by dogs as pack leaders. This experience reinforced in my mind that the training and care of a dog are the responsibilities of adults. Older children can help, but they should never be expected to be solely responsible.

Kids at Training Class

Although I never repeated my Summer School for Kids and Dogs, I do allow children between the age of eight and eighteen to attend group training classes as long as they have a parent with them. Too many times the parents attempted to drop off the kid and dog at class and then leave. What a great deal: dog and child daycare all rolled into one! I quickly informed these parents that they had to stay. The children were allowed to participate and to try training techniques, but only after the parent had mastered them.

Adopted Dog Concerns

As I discuss in other chapters of this book, adolescent and adult dogs often do not pose the same training challenges that puppies do. Many adult dogs have calmed down and have outgrown the mouthing stage.

They are housebroken. They are not evaluating their own sense of dominance. Many older dogs are even intuitively gentle with small children.

On the other hand, some adult dogs do not like children at all. Although I have occasionally met puppies that came into a household not liking children, most dogs that hate kids have learned to do so.

In fact, many adult dogs sitting in shelters have been given away because they bit (or tried to bite) a kid in a previous family. The dog may have been taunted and teased by children or teenagers. A child may have hit or physically abused the dog in some other way. Or the dog may not have been socialized well and was intimidated or frightened of youngsters.

Most times we never know what happened. If you have children in your home and want to adopt a dog, always inquire about a dog's history, especially regarding the dog's experiences with children. Otherwise you are taking a chance with the kids' safety.

If Your Dog Bites

I love dogs. They have been an integral part of my life for many decades, both professionally and privately. I could not fathom living without a dog, even for a day. Nevertheless, I would not own any dog that was a physical threat to my child.

I did not suddenly develop this point of view after having a daughter of my own. I have always believed that the safety of children in a household is more important than owning any specific dog. If you adopted a dog that is growling or snapping at your children, you have the wrong dog.

Is Training the Solution?

Obedience training has the wonderful potential of eradicating many behavioral problems in dogs. Of course, the age of the dog and the type of problem will strongly influence the chance for success. For example, if your adopted dog is a puppy under the age of five months, the prognosis is pretty good that mouthing and some tough-guy aggressive behavior with children can be eliminated. The older the puppy or dog, the worse the success rate becomes.

If I adopted a puppy that showed signs of aggression toward children, I would be more inclined to give training a chance than I would with an adolescent or older dog.

No one can reliably guarantee a dog's behavior, of course, even after training. Do not take a chance with a child's safety by attempting to save a questionable dog. There are too many unwanted dogs that have wonderful temperaments and that are great with kids.

How Children Interact with Dogs

A dog owner once called me looking for help with her two-year-old Airedale terrier. The dog had bitten her three-year-old son on the side of the face. The unfortunate child needed eighteen stitches to close the wound.

After asking this owner a series of questions about the dog and his behavior, I advised her to find another home for the dog. She objected, "No, no, no! This was not the dog's fault. My son deserved it. He put a chesspiece in the dog's ear."

Granted, this child's behavior toward the dog was not right. However, I do not care what kind of dumb thing a preschooler might do to a dog, the child does not "deserve" to be bitten.

Dogs have three options when they are hurt or feel threatened. They can submit and accept whatever is happening to them. They can choose flight and run away. Or they can become aggressive and attack. Regardless of what a child does, the dog must choose one of the first two options—if he is going to remain a member of my family. I urge you to think the same way.

Zero Tolerance Policy

Essentially, I have a zero tolerance policy toward dogs that bite children. But I also have zero tolerance for children who mistreat animals. Toddlers and preschoolers are certainly capable of hurting a dog, however innocently. That's because they are inexperienced and unpredictable. Because of this they should never (I mean never!) be left unsupervised with any dog. I don't care if you own Lassie.

The sweetest, gentlest canine soul I have ever known was our late, great black Labrador retriever, Byron. Byron loved everybody. He kissed bunnies. However, we never left our toddler daughter alone with Byron for two minutes. His seventy-five-pound-body could have unintentionally knocked her over, just as her curious, exploratory nature could have caused him unintended harm. This is one of the big reasons that dogs and small children are so much work. Life becomes a job of nonstop supervision.

Kids need to learn early in life how to interact properly with dogs. These interactions need to be repeated consistently throughout their grade-school years so that they can be caring and responsible pet owners. Every parent has this important obligation.

I have read that children under the age of six do not fully comprehend that animals are living creatures that can feel hurt and pain. Mistreatment by children can cause aggression in dogs, and unfortunately, many dogs end up in shelters because of this aggression. This is the fault of the parents of those children.

Older Children Who Hurt Dogs

I am not a child psychologist. However, I believe that older kids who mistreat animals have a serious emotional and/or psychological problem. I can't even bear to think about some of the horrors that appear in the news from time to time about animal torture and killing. In my opinion, children or teens who do such things don't "outgrow" these tendencies. They need professional help, and they need to be kept away from all animals. If someone in your family or neighborhood fits this description, don't be afraid to speak up about the problem. And keep your pets out of this person's reach.

Proper Play

Playful kids and dogs can sometimes get out of control. Youthful exuberance, competition, and canine dominance have the potential for stirring up problems. Roughhouse play, such as wrestling on the ground or games of tug-of-war that stimulate aggression, should never be allowed. If kids want to play with the dog, they should choose constructive play.

Dogs that love to play "Fetch" or "Find It" make great play companions for children. These are described, along with other fun games, in Chapter 27, "Exercise Is a Must." Kids can even do something as simple as putting the dog on a leash and running around the house twenty-two times. This makes for tired kids and dogs. Both are a good thing!

Other Tips

If you are working through any food-related aggression problems with your adopted dog (described in Chapter 12), be sure that your children are not involved. Children should not have access to such a dog during his mealtimes. Close doors, put up baby gates, or literally stand guard while the dog eats. One mistake could be disastrous. And as I have said before, think long and hard about keeping such a dog in a household with children.

Leash walks with the family dog can be fun for little kids, but an adult needs to go along. Even as a four-year-old, my daughter begged me to let her take our springer spaniel, Crea, out for a walk. Crea is a good leash-walker, and she is always gentle with children. But I never let the two of them go alone. I always anticipated the unpredictable: a stray dog picking a fight, the leash slipping out of her hand, etc. Little kids are not strong enough, dominant enough, or mature enough to handle many kinds of situations. But my daughter certainly could be the one to hold Crea's leash as the three of us strolled down the street. It's just that she has a safety net, in the shape of her dad.

Happily Ever After

If you find the right dog for your family—and your kids are old enough to appreciate and help with dog ownership—it will be a wonderful experience. They will look back fondly on the beloved family dog, and he may be part of their best childhood memories. Because of your efforts, your children will bring good dog-handling skills and caring, responsible attitudes with them to adulthood. And they will be equipped to pass those qualities on to *their* children. You may touch several generations! All because you took the time to treat one adopted dog right.

Chapter 30

Your Adopted Dog and Other Pets

Many dog owners have more than one family pet. Most typically, Rover shares the house with another dog or a cat—or with several of each. It's also possible that he lives with birds, domestic rodents, or reptiles. If your home is virtually a miniature zoo, this chapter may not address your unusual concerns about adopted dogs and exotic animals. But if you need some guidelines about Rover and his more common animal housemates, this chapter will help.

Adding a New Dog to the Pack

If you already own a dog and are thinking about bringing an adopted dog into your home, here are a few guidelines to make things go smoothly. First, be prepared to be a good pack leader. Harmonious packs have strong leaders who do not tolerate fighting and chaos. If you have never owned more than one dog before, reread Chapter 7, "Taking Charge." It will help you think and act like the one who's in control.

Boy meets girl; girl meets boy

The prognosis for harmony in your pack is very good when the new dog is the opposite sex of your resident dog. It is not impossible that a male and female won't get along, but it is unusual.

A resident older male dog will be much more tolerant and accepting of a younger female dog than of another male. That's because when young male dogs join a new pack, they are often inclined to challenge the pack status of an existing male.

If the new dog is more dominant by nature than the resident dog, you are bound to have tension. The newcomer will continue to challenge until he feels that he is in charge. Because the resident dog was there first and especially if he is older, he will probably fight to maintain his pack position. It goes without saying that dogfights are *not* what you want. They will add chaos to your household and potentially cause injury and high veterinary bills. Fights will also undermine your adoption intentions, ending with the new dog being given up once more.

Female dogs do not seem to fight with each other as often as male dogs do. Unfortunately, when females do get into a fight it is often ugly. With females there seems to be less of the noise and posturing that occur between two males. Female dogs try to hurt each other.

Also, male dogs seem to let bygones be bygones. They may get into a horrendous battle and then be okay with each other for days, weeks, or even months—until something sets them off again.

Female dogs often hold grudges. I remember a client who owned two female cocker spaniels. They were sisters from different litters that were about two years apart in age. When the younger dog was about a year old, they got into a nasty fight over a dog toy. From that day on, these two dogs could not look at each other without tearing into one another. The owners ended up placing the younger dog with their adult daughter, who lived across town. Things worked out well. The dogs both ended up in loving homes. But needless to say, they were never invited to join each other for holiday dinners!

An older female resident dog may snap and snarl to let a new male adoptee know who's in charge. But chances are good that she will not attack with the intensity that she would another female dog. Also, most new and younger males quickly learn to be reverent to the queen.

How to make introductions

The best way to introduce adult dogs to each other is off-leash. Being confined to a leash creates dynamics that can lead to a snap, bite, or even a fight. Your resident dog or the new adoptee may feel threatened if he is confined to a leash. Without the opportunity to escape, he may feel that his only option is to become aggressive.

A dog on a leash may feel that he needs to protect you when a new dog approaches. Also, owners have a tendency to tighten up on the leash if they anticipate that their dog might snap. Doing this inadvertently changes the body posture of the dog on the leash by pulling his shoulders up. The other dog may incorrectly interpret this as a sign of dominance.

Off-leash dogs have the opportunity to communicate naturally. If one wants to roll over, belly-up, saying, "Accept me, you're in charge!" he can do so without your interference. If flight instinct kicks in, the dog has the option of getting away.

Unless the two dogs are complete marshmallows and love everybody, you should be prepared in case a fight ensues. The best way to break up a dogfight is with water. Have the garden hose or a bucket of cold water close by in case it is needed. *Do not get between two fighting dogs.* If you try to pry two slashing and biting dogs apart, you are going to get bitten. The worse dog bite that I ever saw happened to a bird-dog trainer. He was trying to separate two of his German shorthaired pointers (females) that were fighting. It was an intense brawl, and it taught me never to get between fighting dogs.

Neutral territory

I have successfully introduced most of my new dogs to the resident dogs in my fenced backyard. However, when friends and I wanted to get our dogs together for the first time, we decided that it would be best to meet on neutral territory.

My late Austrian shepherd, Drifter, although well-trained, was somewhat dominant and territorial. He could be a tough guy with other dominant male dogs. Drifter's instinct to protect his territory was also an incentive to pick a fight. A neutral territory eliminated this factor.

Not only does neutral territory reduce tension, it helps dogs make friends. A fun hike in the woods or a romp in the park enhances bonding. Drifter made many canine buddies after getting to know them on neutral territory. Once he accepted a new dog outside his territory, it was never a problem when the dog came to visit at Drifter's house or yard.

Overcoming disappointment

An adopted dog's arrival may not bring tension and potential fights. It may bring depression and moodiness for your resident dog(s). This is not uncommon, especially for dogs that have been the sole focus of your animal love and devotion.

What to do about it? First, determine that you have made a good adoption decision. A resident dog that is unhealthy or elderly may not have the resilience to adjust to a new pack member. But that is the exception to the rule. Dogs are pack animals, and are usually capable of accepting changes in their pack.

Here are some important guidelines:

Be sure that you are a good pack leader. This provides stability and security to the pack. Don't ignore the first dog in favor of the newcomer. Reserve some individual time and attention for each. Don't reinforce the resident dog's sadness or disappointment with soothing words or petting. Unlike humans who are comforted by such actions, dogs interpret this as praise. Better to say nothing when the "blues" seem to strike.

Fight the blues with fun. Dogs that spend time together doing enjoyable things learn to accept each other more readily. Off-leash hikes, adventurous leash walks, and even side-by-side obedience practice can infuse some happiness and camaraderie into a pack. The tips in Chapter 8, "Bonding from Day One," will give you more ideas for working through the transition.

And give it time. Although some dogs accept a new pack member the day he arrives, others may take days or weeks to adjust. As long as you are attentive, loving, and in charge, your mopey Prince (or Princess) will come around.

Extreme old age

If your resident dog is ten years old or older, I suggest giving serious thought before adding a new dog to the family. This is because old dogs generally are not really tolerant of energetic adolescents that want to jump all over them. Also, dogs are very routine-oriented and may find change difficult to deal with at this time in their lives. It can be very stressful both physically and emotionally for geriatric dogs to deal with a new dog in the family.

Of course, there are exceptions to every rule. It is true that age is subjective to individuals. Some dogs at ten are still in good physical heath and are almost as playful as puppies. Others (especially giant breeds) may be on borrowed time, living well beyond their expected life span.

The personality of your adopted dog is a factor that will influence his ability to live respectfully with a canine senior citizen. If you adopt a dog that is mature and not inclined to pester your elderly dog, there may be no problems. In some cases I've had owners tell me that adding a younger dog to the family was the best thing to happen to old Codger. "He was becoming a couch potato. The new dog now has him playing as he did when he was young." I love hearing that, but it doesn't always work out that way. As you know by now, all dogs are different. Consider how the old guy will react before you adopt.

Cats

One of the many things I admire about humane societies is that they try to collect "cat information" about their adoptable dogs. Did the dog live with a cat? Does he seem to like cats? Does he hate or even kill cats? Adoption workers know that many animal lovers own cats and that a dog adopted into those homes will need to coexist peacefully with the cat—if the dog is to stay.

As I have advised throughout this book, choose your adopted dog wisely. A dog that has had lots of positive cat experiences will have a good chance of doing fine in your home. As a general guideline, I would tend to avoid adopting a stray dog into a cat home, especially if

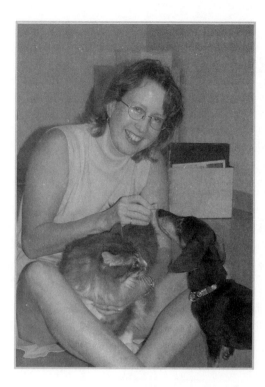

Many adopted dogs previously lived with cats and will probably get along with your own felines. If possible, ask about a dog's "cat experience" before the adoption, and give the cat time and space to adjust to the newcomer.

the dog was a known wanderer. Most wild cats run from dogs. This reinforces a dog's predator-prey feelings toward cats and may put your indoor, pampered feline at risk.

It will come as no surprise to cat lovers that the cat's personality has a lot to do with successful dog-cat relations. We all have met cats that were afraid of people, let alone dogs. Other cats are perfectly calm around dogs and are even interested in them. Our young gray tiger cat, Neville, has a few spaniel friends and has even walked right up to our neighbor's golden retriever puppy to check her out. He sleeps near my own dog, Crea, and occasionally wrestles playfully with her. Neville even willingly submits to "dog baths," a thorough head-licking and ear-cleaning from Crea. Lucky cat. Yuck.

Introduce your adopted dog to your cat (or cats) with minimal fanfare. A quiet house and your calm demeanor will set a peaceful tone. Clip your dog to a leash to avoid unexpected lunging or chasing. Be sure that the cat can jump to safety if needed.

Don't be afraid to correct your cat or your dog if either acts aggressively toward the other. You can even hold a spray bottle filled with plain water (the kind for spraying plants) and direct a spray at either pet if it starts to act aggressively. Your goal is to communicate that hostile behavior will not be tolerated in your home.

If your dog and cat are extremely nervous or agitated around each other, keep them separated for a few days until their individual smells become more familiar around your house. Scent clues are important to animals and will help your dog and cat to understand that both of them belong there with you.

Cats are naturally curious creatures and will sooner or later want to check out the newcomer to the household. If you are crate-training your adopted dog, your cat may take the opportunity to check out the dog while he is safely behind bars in the crate. This is fine and will help both animals become accustomed to each other.

If you have children, remind them not to interfere as the dog and cat get to know each other. Kids can add too much excitement to this situation, which should be a calm one. And you don't want your child hurt if the dog and cat decide to fight or even to play roughly. Teeth and nails can cause a lot of damage.

If you have specific dog-and-cat problems not covered by these general guidelines, speak to your adoption counselor. These individuals handle many, many dogs and cats and have heard hundreds of anecdotes about successful cohabitation. They also know the warning signs when pets are in danger. They can give you useful tips for working through many kinds of difficulties.

A Few Words about Birds

I have some great memories of a cockatiel that I once briefly owned, sitting calmly on my golden retriever Woody's head. Woody's eyes were rolled upward trying to see the bird. To his credit, Woody perfectly obeyed my Sit-Stay command.

I also have a friend who lost two beloved little parrots when they flew out of the bird room and into her terriers' space.

Can birds and dogs coexist? Yes and no, as my two examples demonstrate. Safety for both animals is important. An aggressive bird can give a painful bite. And a dog that is so inclined can kill a bird.

Be sure to know your dogs and birds well before you allow any interaction between them. I knew that the cockatiel was sweet-natured and calm. Woody was obedient and not afraid of new things. Would I let my springer spaniel, Crea, around a pet bird? I strongly doubt it, considering that she's a pheasant-finding machine when we go out hunting. But Byron, our late, great black Lab, could easily have had a lineup of parakeets down his back.

So use your common sense. If you know that your adopted dog once lived with birds, maybe Rover and Tweetie can get to know each other. If in doubt, keep them safely away from each other. Don't let your urge to "see what happens" put any of your pets at risk. It's not worth it.

Domestic Rodents

Terrier owners beware! Your dog was selectively bred to find and kill rodents and other small mammals. In fact, the name "terrier" comes from the Latin word *terra*, meaning "earth." Many terriers earn their keep as "ratters" in horse barns. Other breeds also love this task.

Can you adopt a dog if you (or your kids) keep one or more rodents as pets? Yes, as long as common sense and safety are part of the equation. I would never give a dog unsupervised access to the rodent's cage—or even to the room where the cage is kept. Given enough time and opportunity, many dogs could knock over and open a lightweight cage. At best, the poor rodent gets terrorized. At worst, you come home to one less pet.

I don't doubt that some dog owners have had successful dog-rodent experiences. However, I think these are exceptions to the rule, because dogs are predators by nature. In the wild, rodents are food for canines. If I owned a pet mouse or hamster or guinea pig, I would keep it permanently separated from my dog. These pets can share a house, but I feel that it would be an unnecessary risk to allow them to share the same room.

Chapter 31

Spaying and Neutering Myths

FEW OWNERS OF ADOPTED dogs are unaware of dog overpopulation and why it exists: indiscriminate and excessive breeding. Statistics show that two to three million dogs are killed every year in the United States because they are unwanted. This is a terrible reflection on how we care for and control our domestic dog population. Add to that several million unwanted cats and you can appreciate the sorry mess we have created.

No one person or organization can fix this overwhelming problem. But *every* animal-loving person and organization can contribute in some way. The best place to start is by spaying or neutering all of your pets. Schedule the appointment today.

If your adopted dog came to you from a humane shelter or a breed rescue organization, the dog is probably spayed or neutered already. Don't have any regrets that you cannot breed your dog, even if you think he is a wonderful dog and you want another dog just like him. Keep in mind that everyone thinks their dog is wonderful. Imagine the greater overpopulation mess we would be in if we all bred our dogs simply because we thought they were "wonderful." If you want more dogs in your family, adopt again and socialize, exercise, and train that dog to be wonderful, too. A lot of potential wonderfulness is put to death every year when those two to three million dogs are euthanized.

If your adopted dog is not spayed or neutered, or you are confused as to what is fact and what is myth regarding these procedures, this chapter will help you. Please share it with a friend, too, if you know anyone who needs more information about this topic. The fewer puppies we produce, the closer we are to the day when every dog has a home and an owner who wants him. It may not happen in my lifetime or yours, but every step toward that goal means less killing and less waste of life. That is a worthy goal indeed.

Will Spaying or Neutering Make My Dog Fat?

It is true that there is a tendency for dogs that are spayed or neutered to put on a little weight. But it is really the lack of exercise, too much food at mealtimes, and an endless stream of dog cookies that cause most dogs to become fat. I have met hundreds of overweight dogs whose owners blamed the spaying or neutering surgery for their pets' obesity. It was easier than admitting that they overfed and underexercised their dogs.

Your spayed or neutered dog does not have to become overweight. Food volume and exercise can control body fat. For example, an intact (not neutered) male dog that eats two cups of dry dog food a day may need only a cup and a half to maintain his proper weight after neutering. Certainly his level of exercise, breed, and overall health will influence this food amount, too. Your veterinarian can guide you on specific adjustments with feeding.

A dog that is already overweight can (and should) slim down. The dog's diet might include low-calorie varieties of kibble or special canned food from the vet. This diet can be supplemented with low-calorie items, such as grated carrots, which will add bulk to a meal and provide fiber, vitamins, and minerals.

Every dog that I have ever owned has been spayed or neutered. Not one was ever fat. The only time that they ever started to get chubby was when I became lax with diet and exercise. If I saw them getting a little thick around the middle, I knew it was time to say, "Come on, Crea, we are going for a walk." The best part was that I would lose a few pounds, too.

Will My Dog's Personality Change?

Based on my many experiences living with and knowing lots of spayed and neutered dogs, the only personality changes that I have observed are good ones. Spaying and neutering remove reproductive power, so this surgery only affects sexually oriented behaviors.

I cannot think of one bad reason to lower a dog's sex drive, unless of course you intend to use the dog for breeding. Male dogs in particular have some annoying behaviors that are related to their mating interests.

Neutering is the most effective way to curb these problem behaviors, because obedience training will be undermined by hormones. Testosterone in male dogs is a powerful influence on how the dog acts. Taking this hormone out of the equation improves the success of obedience training.

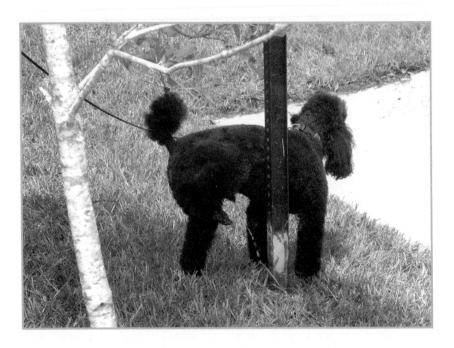

Marking behavior is typical of intact male dogs. If neutered before the behavior develops, many males will never adopt this leg-lift style of urinating.

Marking territory

Intact male dogs are inspired by their sex drive to mark territory, both indoors and out. They do this by lifting their hind leg and releasing urine. Bushes, trees, fence posts, and fire hydrants are all outdoor targets. So are garden tools, swing sets, lawn furniture, and bicycles. Indoors, I have seen dogs mark on sofas, chairs, doorframes, dog beds, human beds—you name it, they'll pee on it.

Leash walks and dog hikes are continuously interrupted by an intact male dog's obsession with urinating on every object along the way.

When a male puppy is neutered before he ever starts to lift his leg, this marking behavior almost never develops. When an older puppy or adult dog is neutered, his marking behavior may diminish, but there is no guarantee that the behavior will be extinguished.

Roaming

Intact male dogs often wander off and roam the neighborhood in order to leave their urinary calling cards. Of course, dogs are always interested in collecting scent information about each other, but sexually motivated dogs can be obsessed. "Who is out there? Are there any females? Are they in heat? Are there any males tougher than me?" We can only guess the extent of what dogs actually can find out about others through their noses.

The urge to mark territory is not the only reason that a male dog may roam. Dogs, by nature, are roving hunters. But marking territory and finding mates are certainly contributing factors. This applies to females, too. A female dog in estrus (heat) is powerfully motivated to be bred. She has a strong urge to seek out mates and will roam far and wide to find them.

After being spayed and neutered, many wandering canines stick closer to home. If contained in a fenced yard, these dogs generally are not obsessed with trying to escape. Their focus is on you, your family, your home, and your routines—not on the opposite sex.

Mounting

Intact male dogs mount females during mating. Unfortunately, they also may mount people's legs or small children when they are sexually frustrated or acting dominant. Needless to say, this behavior is annoying and unacceptable.

A quick and firm correction can often convince most dogs that this behavior will not be tolerated. However, children and even some adults are not capable of delivering an appropriate correction. These individuals are at the mercy of a determined, male dog. Neutering can help to curb this behavior.

Unfortunately, neutering is not a cure-all for some mounting problems. Any dominant dog—male or female, spayed or neutered or not—may use mounting behavior to try asserting dominance. This may be over another dog or over a person. I don't have a problem with dogs sorting out their dominance issues with each other, as long as it does not escalate into a fight. What I don't want to see is a dog trying to mount people. Always correct this behavior in your dog with a growl—"Nhaa!" In addition, clip on the dog's leash and make him do a Down-Stay. He can't annoy you or your friends while lying down and staying in place. Plus, he will be getting a much-needed reminder that he is not the dominant one in the group. You are.

Aggression

I have been a dog professional long enough to know that testosterone is at the root of problem aggression in many dogs. Intact males are more prone to go looking for trouble, such as starting dogfights or attacking defenseless dogs or children.

Canine aggression should never be taken lightly, because the potential for serious harm is too great. Fortunately, dog owners are increasingly held accountable in our courts for any injury or destruction caused by their pets. This is fine with me. I have always believed that we are fully responsible for our pets. Keep the odds in your favor that your dog will never hurt another animal or a person. Spaying and neutering can make a big difference.

Myth: Kids Should Witness the Miracle of Birth

Every year dogs and cats are bred so that children can observe an animal giving birth. Well-intentioned parents do this because they believe they are providing their children with a valuable life experience. But what about teaching kids the bigger picture—of pet overpopulation?

Parents who care about their children should also be concerned with the world that they are handing down to their kids. I hope that today's children will not inherit a world where millions of unwanted pets are killed every year. I believe that children should learn the many ramifications of indiscriminate breeding and the pet overpopulation problem that exists in our society. Teaching a child to be a lifelong responsible pet owner and a champion to the cause of spaying and neutering is far more important than watching Sassy have a litter of pups.

Besides, there are many other ways that children can observe the miracle of birth. Educational videos show animals being born. In rural communities you may be able to visit a farm and watch a foal or calf being born. Just this past year at the Martin County Fair in Stuart, Florida, a mother goat gave birth in the animal display area. It was a neat experience for many people, and my family got to see the little goat when it was just three hours old. We even know one family that allowed their child in the delivery room when the mother gave birth to their second child. So birth is everywhere. It doesn't need to be in your house at the expense of your pets.

Myth: I Cannot Afford the Surgery

Don't let this stop you. Animal welfare organizations of every size have programs to help defer the costs of spaying and neutering. Licensed veterinarians often donate their services. Some programs even offer spaying and neutering for free to anyone who applies, no matter what his or her economic status. It doesn't even matter if the dog was adopted or not. This is a testimony to the importance of spaying and neutering in solving our pet overpopulation problem. Animal advocates want to prevent future killing. You should, too.

Myth: Dogs Should Be Bred for Health Reasons

Veterinary studies have shown that older, unspayed female dogs have a much higher incidence of breast cancer than do spayed females. This is partly because the growth of breast tissue is inhibited when dogs are spayed before the first heat cycle.

Unspayed female dogs also face the risk of pyometra, a life-threatening infection in the uterus. Without emergency veterinary care, a dog with pyometra can die. In most cases, an emergency hysterectomy is performed, and the dog ends up spayed anyway. Better to schedule the surgery when good health, youth, and lack of infection make it a simple, nonthreatening procedure.

The female heat cycle

If helping the canine overpopulation problem and giving your dog a better chance for a healthy life are not good enough reasons for spaying, consider this. Until your female dog is spayed, twice a year you will be dealing with her heat cycle.

Sometime after the dog is six months old, she will come into heat, or estrus. This cycle lasts three weeks. Throughout that time she will bleed, possibly all over your house. Doggie diapers are usually necessary to minimize the mess.

For approximately three days during the heat cycle, the dog will ovulate and will be able to become impregnated. Intact male dogs find this irresistible. Fortunately, experienced males will show interest in the female only during these three days. Because we don't know when those three days occur, the female must never be allowed outside unsupervised during her entire heat cycle.

Unfortunately, unsophisticated males are fascinated by the whole estrus phenomenon. Male suitors of all shapes and sizes will hang around the home of a female dog in heat for weeks on end, creating a disturbance. I heard about one determined terrier that lay motionless—for days—under a garden bush near a female golden retriever's front door. Rain, darkness, cold, hunger, and other male dogs could not drive this little dog away. Neither could the golden's annoyed owners. After spaying their dog later that year, they never saw the terrier again. I'd like to think that he was safely fenced in or perhaps was neutered, but he probably just moved on to more "fertile" hunting grounds.

Male health benefits

Intact male dogs have a higher percentage of medical problems than neutered males. Testicular and prostate cancer are two serious diseases seen in older intact males. These and other ailments can be avoided if male dogs are neutered before problems arise.

"I Wouldn't Want Someone to Do That to Me!"

Many male dogs are not neutered because their male owners cringe at the thought of it. "I could never do that to Rocco. He'd turn into a wimp." Nothing can be further from the truth. I have owned neutered male dogs that were stellar athletes. They could swim, run, and hunt as well as any intact male.

Neutering also does not diminish a dog's protective instinct in the least. An adult male dog that is bonded to his family and his home will almost always have an urge to guard them. Some of my neutered male dogs would ferociously protect me, my home, and my car from anyone they did not know. Testicles or not, these dogs were wary and tough.

If a man is reluctant to neuter his male dog because he wouldn't want "someone to do that to him," he should look at his dog's life realistically. If an intact male dog is never allowed to mate, it is natural that he will become sexually frustrated. He will spend his entire existence with no sexual release. This frustration is bound to manifest itself in behaviors that humans consider unacceptable. The marking, roaming, mounting, and aggression described above are just some of the problems that an intact male can create for his owners. And owners of unspayed females get the responsibility and expense of health care for a mother and her puppies, the turmoil of a houseful of canine young-sters, and the difficulty of finding responsible owners for all the pups. I really can't think of any good reason at all to avoid spaying or neu-tering a pet. If this chapter has not convinced you, nothing will. I'm sorry to say that you remain part of the problem. I sincerely hope you change your mind.

Epilogue

Giving Back—
More Ways to Help
Unwanted Dogs

WITH THE HELP OF THIS BOOK, you and your adopted dog have a long and happy future in front of you. Your efforts with one dog have put a tiny but meaningful dent in the problem of pet overpopulation. A life was not only saved, it is being enriched with exercise, health care, a good diet, obedience training, and love. You deserve the thanks of anyone who cares about dogs.

Is there more to do? Indeed there is. Consider the various suggestions listed here. Each and every one of them will help homeless animals in some way. Good luck with your ongoing efforts . . . and thank you.

* Adopt your next pet. You learned a lot by adopting and training your current dog. Your experience is valuable and will help another animal succeed. Don't be afraid to do it again. Reread this book if you need help!
* Provide a foster pet home. Some animals need short-term care while they await permanent adoption. This can happen when shelters get too full, when health problems require specialized

handling, or when an animal is in transit to its new owners. Perhaps your fenced backyard and outgrown kennel crate can be put to good use for a few weeks or months. Providing foster care is a great way to help out.

✳ Donate pet-care items. Animal shelters and pounds need food, blankets, towels, and other supplies. By simply spring-cleaning your linen closet or pantry you may fill a bag with useful things. An outgrown kennel crate or training collar, just lying around your garage, can help another adoptable dog get off to a good start. Spare leashes, food bowls, and toys will readily be put to use by any adoption organization.

✳ Donate money, of course. The physical housing of unwanted animals generates electric and heating bills, water and sewer bills, staff payroll expenses, the need to purchase basic supplies, such as food and dog shampoo, the obligation to pay for insurance and taxes, and the responsibility to provide veterinary care. Money is not as personal as other kinds of contributions, but it is essential. Without it, homeless animals would have no place to go.

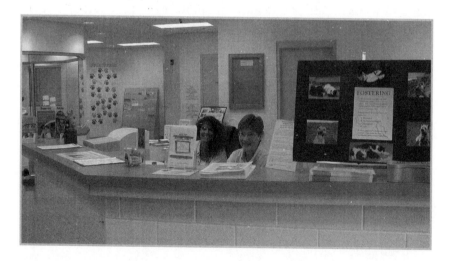

Animal welfare organizations always need our support. You can help by donating money or supplies and by volunteering your time. The organization you help may one day rescue and care for your next adoptable dog!

❋ Go walk a homeless dog. Or cuddle an unwanted cat. Volunteer opportunities abound at animal shelters and humane societies. Even one hour a week of hands-on helping can make a difference. Your efforts can free up busy staff workers when you provide help with paperwork, do cleaning chores, answer the telephones, or do other tasks.

❋ Animal-related duties can be especially rewarding. Your warmth and gentleness can sooth a troubled canine soul. Your energy can be used to inspire exercise and play. Your patience can be put to use teaching leash-walking or other basic obedience skills. Every improvement in every homeless dog's behavior makes that dog more adoptable. Socialization, exercise, and training will help every time.

❋ Vote for the animals. Watch for proposals of animal-friendly legislation in your local or state governments. Or generate your own proposal! Cast your vote to protect animals, and contact your representatives to encourage them to do the same. After you take the time to study animal-related issues, share what you have learned with others. Educate your pet-loving friends so they can vote for the animals, too.

❋ Be an animal advocate. This means speaking up when your neighbor has his dog tied out all night in subzero temperatures. It means reporting neglect or abuse to the police or animal control officer. It means helping an injured pet by the side of the road (as long as you can do so safely). It means helping lost animals reunite with their owners by checking identification tags on strays and calling the owner, paying attention to "lost pet" posters, checking the classified ads for missing animals, and noticing unfamiliar dogs or cats in your neighborhood.

Animal advocates also think of ways to prevent harm to pets. They check for leaks of sweet-tasting but poisonous radiator fluid in their driveways (or replace ordinary fluid with a non-toxic version). They do not set out garbage pails where pets can raid them or leave the pails overnight near a busy roadway. Animal advocates do not let dogs ride in the back of their open pickup trucks. They slow down when an animal, even a wild animal, is near the side of the road and risks being hit. They don't plant harmful shrubs or flowers in their yard or grow poisonous plants in their house.

* Set a good example for your children. Let your animal advocacy be visible to young people. They will learn a lot by your example, and depending on their ages, they can join you in your efforts. Be sure to teach responsible pet care in your home. Explain to your children that owning a pet requires daily feeding, frequent exercising, grooming, obedience training, and trips to the veterinarian. Instruct them to treat all animals with kindness. And let your example of doing so speak even louder than your words.

* Make your own dog an advocate for adoption. Let people know that such an awesome, well-trained animal was once homeless or unwanted. When you walk him around the neighborhood or take him to visit a nursing home or to play fetch with the kids down at the park, you are showing off the joys of an adopted dog. It can remind people how many wonderful animals are waiting for homes and also give them hope that they, too, could end up with such a treasure.

And don't ever be apologetic that your dog is "just a mutt from the pound." If he is a well-behaved, wonderful companion, you have a lot to be proud of—and thankful for. Your dog may have been the lucky one to get adopted, but in the end, you are the lucky one to have the truest kind of friend: a loving and devoted dog.

A Personal Afterword

WHAT A LONG FUN TRIP it's been. This journey started three decades ago, when I began following the New England and Tri-State dog obedience trial circuit. This leg of the trip lasted for seven years. After earning fourteen American Kennel Club obedience titles, I had the "dog bug" imbedded deeply into my soul.

From there the road led me west to sunny Southern California for three years. The dogs were the same as on the East Coast, but the weather was better. Here I had the opportunity to bring together a blend of my two favorite pastimes, fooling around with dogs and beach bumming. I also had a revelation on the West Coast. I was no longer interested in the world of doggie competitions. Helping people to have well-trained pets became my passion. It still is today.

The road then looped its way back east to Connecticut. For seven years I spent six-and-a-half days a week crisscrossing lower Fairfield County, teaching people how to train their dogs. During this time I met my writing partner and wife, Barbara McKinney, and we combined our skills. Barbara is a professional editor and dog enthusiast. (Who would think that four years at Dartmouth College and a graduate degree in journalism would all go to the dogs!) Together Barbara and I developed training programs, wrote magazine articles, and did an hour-long weekly radio show about dogs. We ran at a frenzied pace. We also signed a publishing contract to "get it all down on paper."

The next leg was by boat back to the beach. We were off to

Nantucket Island for a six-month hiatus to write our first book, *Dog Talk: Training Your Dog Through a Canine Point of View*. Six months turned into nine years. Nine remarkable years, during which time we taught islanders how to train their dogs, started writing a weekly newspaper column, wrote two more books, and had a daughter.

We also spread the ashes of three beloved canine family members over their favorite beaches and moors on our island home.

The new millennium and another turn in the road found us on the banks of the Connecticut River in the green mountains of central Vermont. For two years we got to know some Yankee dogs and their owners, on both sides of the river. We even adopted a cat.

Now we have changed latitudes once again. We turned south to the sunshine and subtropical air of southeastern Florida where two wide rivers meet the sea. Here we have completed our fourth book, *Adoptable Dog*.

While gathering information for this project, one of the shelter administrators that we interviewed asked me, "What do you see yourself doing with dogs next?"

I was surprised to find myself without a definitive answer. My life has been a somewhat unconventional one, and I can never really predict which way the wind will blow and where I'll turn up next. I do know that I'll be fooling around with dogs in some interesting way—and probably going to the beach.

—John Ross, with Crea
March 2002
End of the beach at Sailfish Point
Stuart, Florida

Appendix A

Adoptable Dogs on the World Wide Web

THESE ARE JUST A FEW of the websites that provide vast amounts of information about adoptable dogs. On these sites you can search for a dog by breed, age, geographic location, and other variables. Pictures are often included as well. You also can search for all of the adoption organizations in your state or local area, including municipal shelters, humane societies, nonprofit groups, and breed rescue networks.

The adoptable dogs featured on these and similar websites usually have been fully vaccinated, checked for worms and other parasites, and spayed or neutered. Thanks to various sponsors, these dogs also may come with coupons for dog food, certificates for training class, a new leash and collar, and even pet health insurance. There is no chance that you won't find a great adoptable dog through one of the sites, probably waiting for you at a shelter not far from your home. Go online and take a look.

Petfinder.com—extensive search functions for dogs and adoption
    organizations
www.petfinder.com

PetShelter Network—state-by-state listings of almost 2,000 animal shelters
www.petshelter.org

Pets 911—extensive listings of dogs and adoption resources
www.1888pets911.org

1-800-Save-A-Pet.com—search functions for shelters and dogs
www.1-800-save-a-pet.com

DogOMania Dogs in Need—listing many shelters and adoption resources
www.dogomania.com

Senior Canine Rescue Society—specializing in older and senior dogs
www.seniordogrescue.org

Big Paws Rescue—specializing in large and giant breeds
www.bigpawsrescue.tripod.com

American Kennel Club's National Breed Club Rescue Network—listing contact information for breed clubs and many breed rescue groups
www.akc.org/breeds/rescue.cfm

When you are offline: Your local telephone book is also an excellent resource for finding adoption organizations in your area. Check the yellow page listings under headings such as "animal shelters" or "humane societies." Government listings for your city, town, or county can put you in touch with the municipal pound, often listed under animal control, health department, or police department.

Humane Societies

The Humane Society of the United States
2100 L Street, NW
Washington DC 20037
202-452-1100
www.hsus.org

This organization coordinates a vast number of animal protection efforts. The HSUS assists local humane societies, aids in protecting wildlife, helps to protect farm animals, monitors animal-related legislation, provides educational programs, and works to overcome animal cruelty in any setting. The regional offices assist individuals and organizations on many animal-related issues.

Regional Offices

Central States Regional Office
800 West 5th Avenue #110
Naperville, IL 60563
630-357-7015
Fax: 630-357-5725
E-mail: csro@hsus.org

Great Lakes Regional Office
745 Haskins Street
Bowling Green, OH 43402-1696
419-352-5141
Fax: 419-354-5351
E-mail: glro@hsus.org

Mid–Atlantic Regional Office
Bartley Square
270 Route 206
Flanders, NJ 07836
973-927-5611
Fax: 973-927-5617
E-mail: maro@hsus.org

Midwest Regional Office
1515 Linden Street Suite 220
Des Moines, IA 50309
515-283-1393
Fax: 515-283-1407
E-mail: mwro@hsus.org

New England Regional Office
Route 112, Halifax Jacksonville
    Town Line
Mailing address: P.O. Box 619
Jacksonville, VT 05342-0619
802-368-2790
Fax: 802-368-2756
E-mail: nero@hsus.org

Northern Rockies Regional
    Office
490 North 31st Street, Suite 215
Billings, MT 59101
406-255-7161
Fax: 406-255-7162
E-mail: nrro@hsus.org

Pacific Northwest Regional
    Office
5200 University Way NE
    Suite 201
Seattle, WA 98105-3597
206-526-0949
Fax: 206-526-0989
E-mail: pnro@hsus.org

Southeast Regional Office
1624 Metropolitan Circle, Suite B
Tallahassee, FL 32308
850-386-3435
Fax: 850-386-4534
E-mail: sero@hsus.org

Southwest Regional Office
3001 LBJ Freeway, Suite 224
Dallas, TX 75234
972-488-2964
Fax: 972-488-2965
E-mail: swro@hsus.org

West Coast Regional Office
5301 Madison Avenue, Suite 202
Mailing address:
P.O. Box 417220
Sacramento, CA 95841-7220
916-344-1710
Fax: 916-344-1808
E-mail: wcro@hsus.org

Additional Humane Organizations

American Humane Association—
resource for animal and child
welfare
63 Inverness Drive East
Englewood, CO 80112-5117
800-227-4645
303-792-9900
303-792-5333 (fax)
www.americanhumane.org

Spay/USA—resource for low-
cost spaying and neutering
2261 Broadbridge Ave.
Stratford, CT 06614
1-800-248-SPAY
www.spayusa.org

Doris Day Animal League—
supporting humane treatment
of animals
227 Massachusetts Ave., NE,
Suite 100
Washington, D.C. 20002
202-546-1761
www.ddal.org

Best Friends Animal Sanctuary—
one of the nation's largest pet
sanctuaries
5001 Angel Canyon Road
Kanab, UT 84741-5001 USA
Phone: (435) 644-2001
Fax: (435) 644-2078
www.bestfriends.org

Note: To find the many regional and local humane societies found
throughout the United States and Canada, use the resources described in
Appendix A.

Index

Page numbers in *italics* refer to illustrations.

About the Authors

John Ross

Nationally known dog obedience instructor John Ross has been training dogs for thirty years. He is the author of several books, including *Puppy Preschool* and the classic training guide *Dog Talk*. John has earned more then a dozen AKC obedience titles with his own dogs but now focuses strictly on pet training. Since 1994 he has been writing a question-and-answer newspaper column that often is called the "Miss Manners of Dogs."

During his long career, John has taught his popular in-home obedience program in six states. Now based in Florida, he presents talks and workshops for pet owners and continues to teach fundamental obedience. He loves talking about dogs and is glad to provide help to America's 39 million dog owners. He can be reached at dogtalk1@bellsouth.net.

Barbara McKinney

A professional editor and writer since 1979, Barbara McKinney began her involvement with dog obedience training in 1985. She had collaborated with John on all of his published works, including magazine articles, training books, and a weekly newspaper column. She co-wrote the script for his *Puppy Preschool* video and was co-host of their weekly radio show, *Dog Talk*. In 1993 John and Barbara's longtime working partnership became a marriage partnership as well.